ROLL THE DICE, PICK A DOC AND HOPE FOR THE BEST

By

LEN KREISLER MD

Copyright © 2009 Len Kreisler

All rights reserved.
No part of this book may be reproduced or transmitted in any form, by any means (electronic, phoyocopying, recording, or otherwise) without the prior written permission of the author.

ISBN: 1-4392-2332-7
ISBN-13: 9781439223321

Visit www.booksurge.com to order additional copies.

DEDICATION

TO THE TRULY COMMITTED HEALTHCARE WORKERS
TOILING TO PUT THE ODDS IN YOUR FAVOR

SITUATIONS VARY – HUMAN NATURE REMAINS CONSTANT

For those of us who spawned the baby boomers after World War II, we can pleasantly recall the strong bonds between the family doctor and his patients. Dr. Gillespy and Marcus Welby were national icons. Payments were mostly in cash, occasionally in barter or written off. Insurance was either Blue Shield/Blue Cross, or some other program provided by an employer. Medicare and Medicaid were non-existent as we entered the golden age of medicine after WWII. The indigent were taken care of in free clinics funded by state and local agencies.

Few ever thought of suing and malpractice insurance for a family practitioner doing surgery and deliveries was well under a $1000 per year. Today it is between $100,000 and 200,000 per year…or higher…if available.

Governmental intrusions, massive paperwork, managed care, boutique medicine, physician advertising, supermarket walk-in clinics, physician assistants, nurse practitioners and huge office overheads weren't even on the drawing boards. It was not as high tech as today's promotions, but lives were saved and bodies healed. Doctor/patient loyalties took priority to indifference or special interests.

The medical infrastructure has become stretched and fragmented.

What are your odds of getting access to timely, affordable, quality medical care? Do you understand how the game is played? This book may help you appreciate the odds.

THE AUTHOR GRADUATED THE UNIVERSITY OF VERMONT SCHOOL OF MEDICINE IN 1957.
GENERAL ROTATING INTERNSHIP

CAPTAIN U.S. ARMY MEDICAL CORPS
(FT. DETRICK AND FT. RITCHIE)

13 YEARS HOME/OFFICE FAMILY PRACTICE
(PEEKSKILL, N.Y.)

18 YEARS MEDICAL DIRECTOR NEVADA OPERATIONS OFFICE OF THE DEPARTMENT OF ENERGY

CHIEF OF STAFF SOUTHERN NEVADA TEACHING HOSPITAL

4 YEARS CRUISE SHIP PHYSICIAN

SPECIAL TRAINING IN WEAPONS OF MASS DESTRUCTION—BIOLOGICAL AND NUCLEAR

ACTIVIST—ALWAYS

Board certified by the AMA approved boards of specialties in Family Practice and Occupational and Environmental Medicine and certified Medical Review Officer for substance abuse, surveillance and treatment.

Former FAA medical examiner.

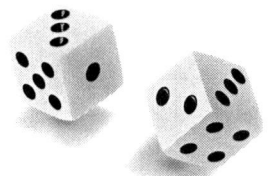 # CHAPTER I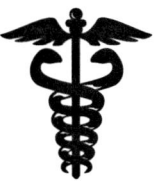

ALL DOCTORS ARE NOT CREATED EQUAL

New acquaintances invariable ask:
"What kind of doctor are you?"
My answer depends on prevailing mood and ambiance.
My response might be: "I'm a real doctor, or, I'm a money doctor."
They smile. "No, really, what is your specialty?" they ask.
I get serious: "I was a Marcus Welby-type family doc for 13 years; home-office practice. I delivered 'em and buried 'em; and everything in between. I even made house calls."
The older generation responds with knowing nostalgia. Others show disappointment. I can read their thoughts: *Just a general practitioner at the lower end of the medical care chain: jack of all trades and master at none.*
I try to bolster my standing. I quickly ad: "I'm also Board certified in Occupational and Environmental Medicine,"
Their facial response varies: frowns, caution, quizzical or just plain blank.

I explain that there are only around 1500 in the United States certified by the American Medical Association's Board of Specialties, and that I was the second M.D. so certified in the state of Nevada in 1980. Currently, Nevada may have 2-3 more. I also explain that the specialty deals with man and his workplace; like air quality, noise levels, medically safe work environments, drugs in the workplace, ergonomics, radiation, chemicals… they get the idea and my status improves.

Then it's my turn to ask questions. Do you know the difference between an Intern and an Internist? Okay, how about an Allopathic doctor (M.D.) and an Osteopathic doctor (D.O.)? Or, Homeopathic, Chiropractic, Podiatric, Naturopathic and others who claim the title "physician." Then I ask about their knowledge of allied health professionals like psychologists (versus psychiatrists), counselors, physician assistants, paramedics, nurse practitioners, therapists and assorted *medical extenders*…who readily accept the title of *DOC*, when conferred by well-meaning but uninformed patients.

The 64-dollar questions relate to training, certification and licensing. Few in the lay public know the facts. National standards may be vague or absent. State rules and regulations vary and the laws that do exist are only as good as the ongoing oversight. The patient, now called the consumer or client, holds the medical dice in their hands; they need to know the facts and the odds on the care they're given, or opt to take.

I'll start with two big categories: Allopathic doctors (M.D.) and Osteopathic doctors (D.O.). Both groups have good apples and bad apples… and important differences.

Andrew H. Beck, Brown Medical School, Providence, RI, wrote an excellent synopsis of 19th and 20th century medical reforms emerging into the current Allopathic disciplines required for an M.D. degree in the United States. THE FLEXNER REPORT AND THE STANDARDIZATION OF AMERICAN MEDICAL EDUCATION; May 5, 2004, student JAMA article.

"In the 19th century, most medical education in the United States was administered through 1 of 3 basic systems: an apprenticeship system, in which students received hands-on instruction from a local practitioner; a proprietary school system, in which groups of students attended a course of lectures from physicians who owned the medical college; or a university system, in which students received some combination of didactic and clinical training at university-affiliated lecture halls and hospitals. These medical schools taught diverse types of medicine, such as scientific, osteopathic, homeopathic, chiropractic, eclectic, physiomedical, botanical, and Thomsonian. In addition, wealthy and industrious medical students supplemented their education with clinical and laboratory training in the hospitals and universities of Europe, primarily in England, Scotland, France and Germany. Because of the heterogeneity of educational experiences and the paucity of licensing examinations, physicians in America at the turn of the 20th century varied tremendously in their medical knowledge, therapeutic philosophies and aptitudes for healing the sick."

Does this sound familiar? Andrew Beck quotes medical educator John Shaw Billings in 1891; "The great mass of the public know little and care less about the details of professional education…The popular feeling is that in a free country everyone should have the right to follow any occupation he likes, and employ for any purpose any one whom he selects, and that each party must take the consequences."

Sounds somewhat like today's professional lobbyist justifying special interest legislation, or a congressional legislator pushing for an earmark (hometown pork). The American Medical Association (AMA) showed vision and determined leadership in 1904 when it created the Council on Medical Education (CME) to promote the restructuring of medical education in the United States. The CME came up with a format of 2 years in basic science training followed by 2 years of clinical training. Has the AMA strayed from its leadership role? Why has M.D. membership in the AMA been under fifty percent of the eligible MD's? Ask your doctor?

    The CME asked Carnegie Foundation president, Henry Pritchett, to help with medical school reform. Mr. Pritchett got schoolmaster and educational theorist, Abraham Flexner, to study the subject and spearhead the drive for educational standards, accountability and licensing. Flexner felt that business ethics were not compatible with progressive academic values: Andrew Beck quotes Flexner;

    "Such exploitation of medical education is strangely inconsistent with the social aspects of medical practice. The overwhelming importance of preventive medicine, sanitation and public health indicates that in modern life the medical profession is an organ differentiated by society for its highest purposes, not a business to be exploited."

Despite many changes and advances, the delivery of health care continues to attract some with exploitation in their souls.

"In 1912, a group of licensing boards formed the Federation of State Medical Boards, which voluntarily agreed to base its accreditation policies on academic standards determined by the AMA's CME. By the 1930's, the combined efforts of state licensing boards, philanthropic foundations, and the AMA's CME, resulted in the eradication of America's proprietary medical colleges and the standardization of the laboratory, and hospital-based research medical university model that Flexner advocated in his report."

According to the Directory of American Medical Education, as of 2005, the United States has 125 allopathic medical schools, i.e. schools granting MD degrees. We have heavily endowed private institutions as well as state schools of medicine, with varying degrees of state funding. For example, my alma mater, The University of Vermont School of Medicine (UVM) receives a relatively small percentage of annual funding from the state, while the University of Nevada School of Medicine (UNSOM) gets the majority of its funding from the state. Funding benefits from philanthropic gifts, endowments and research grants. Older institutions have had more time to develop alternative resources.

Annual tuition at some of the private schools have gone over $40,000, and a significant number of medical graduates get their MD degree with a hefty debt….frequently over $100,000. Details about any of the 125 allopathic schools can be obtained through the Association of American Medical Colleges (AAMC).

The devil is in the details when one talks about 21st century state licensing boards. States can be similar or significantly different. Nevada, for example, has separate licensing boards for MD's and DO's, while Alabama has a combined board (MD and DO) for anyone seeking to get licensed as a physician to practice medicine and surgery in the state of Alabama.

"All, except 14 states have combined boards. Those 14 with separate boards are:

ARIZONA	NEVADA	UTAH
CALIFORNIA	NEW MEXICO	VERMONT
FLORIDA	OKLAHOMA	WASHINGTON
MAINE	PENNSYLVANIA	WEST VIRGINIA
MICHIGAN	TENNESSEE	

NY and IL are unique in that those states have one medical board whose function is to *license* physicians and another board whose function is to *regulate/discipline* physicians. The medical boards in IL fall under the umbrella of the IL Department of Financial and Professional Regulation (data from Federation of State Medical Boards)."

I favor a combined board, which holds all physicians to the same standards and regulations.

In Nevada, The State Board of Medical Examiners (M.D. board) is totally separate from the Nevada Board of Osteopathic Physicians. In my opinion, from 1973 to the present, the D.O. Board has been virtually non-existent when it comes to professional oversight of its members. The M.D. Board has done a better job, but still has glaring deficiencies. The consumer (potential patient) should want to know what's done in their state, and in states where they travel, vacation or do business.

While no medical licensing board, to my knowledge, has a perfect oversight batting average, the Nevada M.D. board has issued timely reprimands, limited license stipulations and license revocations. I'd give it a 75% positive rating. Since 1973 (when I arrived in Nevada), I know of no Osteopathic license revocation, and until recently, there weren't any reprimands or limited license stipulations, to my knowledge. Sometime after 2000, two Nevada Osteopaths got their wrists slapped. One was accused of using animal grade Botox, among other unacceptable things, and the other was accused of causing significant eye damage to at least 12 patients due to substandard eye surgery. Both are still practicing.

In June 2007, the primary Las Vegas newspaper, The Review Journal, reported that the former deputy director of the State Board of Osteopathic Medicine was being investigated as to why patient complaints hadn't been properly investigated. The executive director of the Osteopathic Board stated to the Review Journal that the DO Board had been without sufficient operating funds to have had acceptable administrative investigation into complaints of misconduct and malpractice, for at least the previous two years. If the MD Board needs additional operating funds, it assesses the membership. The DO board could easily do the same. Nevada now has an Osteopathic Medical School located in Henderson, Nevada. You can see why I favor a combined licensing board. Last I heard, their tuition was $30,000 per year. Nevada's state (MD) school is in the neighborhood of $12,000 per year (2007).

As with all licensing bodies, they cannot assign damages for a patient. They can reprimand, modify or revoke a practitioner's license, and they can recover the board's investigative/administrative costs for themselves, but nothing for the patient. If the patient wants to seek damages, they need to hire a lawyer and go to civil or criminal court.

Most boards are selected from names submitted to the Governor. In Nevada, as elsewhere, *JUICE* plays an important role in the selection process. As with real juice, the quality of the end product has a lot to do with the starting quality of fruits and vegetables going into the mix. Interesting debates occur over appointed bodies versus other methods of selection. It's a roll of the dice: sometimes we hit a winning streak, regardless of the process used.

When a Board renders an opinion, the physician may appeal the decision to a judge, all the way to the state supreme court. However, as stated, if the plaintiff-patient seeks damages, they must hire a lawyer and go to court on their own. The patient may challenge the Board's decision with respect to its findings about a licensed practitioner, but the Board's ruling is final and will stand. That decision has no appeal for the plaintiff/patient and only the Governor could intercede….fat chance.

As of 2007, the United States has 23 Osteopathic medical schools (MedSchoolReady.com). The DO's have the same rights and privileges as the

MD's, but there are differences above and beyond licensing: i.e. philosophy, research, entrance requirements, training and oversight. Quoting from the same dot com: "Osteopathic (DO) medical schools are somewhat easier to get into than allopathic (MD) medical schools due to lower average GPA and MCAT requirements. However, admission to osteopathic medical schools is still competitive. Generally speaking, most osteopathic schools do not have large local teaching hospitals affiliated with them. In fact, in some cases, core (and often other) 3rd and 4th year rotations are not locally offered at all. Some countries, outside the U.S., do not recognize DO medical degrees.

With respect to residency; i.e. postgraduate specialty training: "DO graduates can apply for both (DO) residencies (from which MD applicants are precluded) and allopathic (MD) residencies in all specialties, but may find it slightly harder to compete with MD's for allopathic (MD) residencies. Some very competitive MD residency programs are virtually impossible for osteopathic graduates to get into."

The following quote from IMU (InterAmerican Medical University: medschoolready.com) will no doubt bring a lot of complaints. I strongly agree with the characterizations. If the reader has problems with it, they should e-mail IMU directly.

"What distinguishes the osteopathic (DO) medical schools slightly from allopathic (MD) medical schools is the osteopathic philosophy or approach to medicine. Besides the normal basic science and clinical curriculum, DO students also learn Osteopathic Manipulation (referred to as OMM or OTM most of the time), which comes close to a cross between physical therapy and chiropractic—it's really neither, because it is unique in its own right, but address some of the same type of musculoskeletal problems as the two professions mentioned."

Physical therapy and chiropractic have their own licensing boards and I'll address those, and others, shortly. If the reader wants a factual, critical treatise on Osteopathy, I would recommend reading:

DUBIUOS ASPECTS OF OSTEOPATHY
By
Stephen Barrett, M.D.
http://www.quackwatch.org

Dr. Barrett, on page 2, hits the nail on the head: "However, as with (all) medical graduates, the quality of individual graduates depends on how bright they are, how hard they work, and what training they get after graduation. Those who diligently apply themselves can emerge as competent."

I would add that hopefully, all those seeking the title of physician will abide by acceptable moral and ethical values.

My position on Oriental Medicine, Chiropractic and Faith Healing is this: they rely heavily on the placebo effect; i.e. tell someone something will help and at least 30% will report that it did help. The science is shaky or absent to justify the claims of those practitioners. Insurance payments, private or governmental, should not be allowed. That alone would make patients think twice about seeking that type of service. In addition:

1. Medical diagnoses by any of those entities should be critically reviewed for acceptable accuracy, and prosecuted if found to be scientifically unsubstantiated. This represents incompetence and/or fraud.
2. Those practitioners should not be allowed to do their own radiological examinations, nor should they be allowed to order, or use, radiographic examinations done by licensed specialists completing allopathic (MD) residencies.

3. Those 3 groups of practitioners are already prohibited from writing for prescription medications. They do use over the counter products and imported concoctions that carry risks of dangerous drug interactions as well as direct adverse health effects. Health supplements and over the counter remedies have been found to contain hormones, tranquilizers, stimulants, and other unacceptable items. The FDA (Food and Drug Administration) should be given unfettered authority to police these areas (which it currently lacks), and appropriate oversight to see that violators are prosecuted with meaningful penalties.

I'm sure patients, practitioners and product suppliers will go ballistic with the above. However, those are my professional opinions, and I welcome open, public debate in a neutral forum. I will discuss pharmaceuticals, supplements and the FDA in a separate chapter.

We have entered the 21st century with new buzzwords for health care delivery: boutique medicine and walk-in clinics are among the latest entrepreneurial promotions. Supply, demand and economics leads to creativity. Health care demands and patient expectations keep going up. Well- trained practitioners struggle with rising volume and burdensome re-embursement. Accountability becomes an afterthought or disappears…and the gross national happiness product varies with the patient's socio-economic status. Politicians roll the dice and support the best odds for re-election, rather than learning the best health care options and legislating for the greater good. Let's look at case examples:

When I was Medical Director for the Atomic Test Program in Nevada, I invited physicians, allied health professionals and their significant others, to tour the Nevada Test Site. We spent the day educating the visitors on the Department of Energy's mission and accomplishments at the Nevada Test Site, and the medical program for its workers and their families. One government employee asked if I could invite Dr. Wong MD CM (not his real name). The employee was certain his Dr. Wong was a medical doctor. However, I had never seen "MD CM" so I called his office and found it stood for, "Medical Doctor Chinese Medicine."

Asian Medicine (in Nevada) has its own licensing board and I was told it was created during a legislative session by inviting the legislators to a storefront demonstration across from the capitol building…lobbying at its finest. I further discovered that Dr. Wong was previously a card dealer at a local hotel/casino with no details on how he qualified to practice Oriental Medicine. I tried calling the number listed in the phone book and got a recording that the number was no longer in operation. An ad in the yellow pages for a practitioner of Oriental Medicine reads as follows:

SPECIALIZING IN PAIN CONTROL AND HERBAL MEDICINE

- **Arthritis-Tics-Stroke-Tennis elbow-Weight-Emotional**
- **Bursitis-Emphysema-Sciatica-Lumbago-Smoking Control**
- **Sinusitis-Psoriasis-Neuritis-Tremor-Baldness**
- **Migraine-Whiplash-Neuralgia-Shingles-Facelift**
- **Asthma-Strain-Tendonitis-Spastic Colon-Prostate/Sex**
- **Allergy-Muscle-Spasm-Gout-Nerve Deafness-Tinnitus and skin problems. The ad goes on to offer electric or traditional acupuncture, as well as *Moxibustion* and *Acusuction* (I assume the latter is a form of ancient cupping to draw out the "poisons" in your body)."**
- **Worker's Compensation-Auto Accidents**
- **Other insurance cases considered**

In my opinion, Oriental Medicine should not be given eligibility for insurance reembursement, nor should they be allowed to take Worker's Compensation cases. I see no credibility to their philosophy, training and therapeutic claims. If you see otherwise, I have a bridge in Brooklyn for sale…cheap.

Keep in mind, many of these alternative health care promoters use worthless, often dangerous, food supplements and herbs…. not supervised by the Food and Drug Administration. Here's an example of playing Russian Roulette with what goes into your mouth.

In 1980, I completed the pre-requisites, including a mini-residency, and was allowed to take the two-day examination for the specialty of Occupational and Environmental Medicine. I was the second person so certified in the state of Nevada by the allopathic (MD) board of specialties. There were approximately 1200 nationwide at the time, and maybe an additional 300 after 2000. Occupational and Environmental Medicine deals with man and his environment—occupational settings, activities of daily living and recreational pursuits. Areas like sound, air quality, ergonomics, water quality, carcinogens, exposure to energy waves of the entire spectrum, work-specific hazards, promoting safety and health, drug surveillance and rehabilitation, food production, sanitation, public health, aerospace medicine …to give you a general idea of the wide scope of this specialty. Worker's Compensation is a high priority area.

Many worker's compensation cases are unquestionably valid, while others are clearly at the other end of the spectrum. The gray areas in the middle of the spectrum are often difficult and complex. My position has always been in favor of the worker in cases of unclear causation. It becomes more problematic when practitioners with questionable credentials gain credibility through misguided political and court recognition. It creates false legitimacy to a claim. Consider this case:

A man worked as a carpenter at the Nevada Test Site for 10 years. His medical records revealed normal, very complete annual physical examinations in accordance with the Department of Energy rules and regulations. No history of any work related injuries. He retired to Texas at age 60. Three years after leaving the Test Site, he files a worker's compensation claim, from Texas, for three collapsed vertebrae in his lower back. He claimed (with his out of state medical documentation) that repetitive motion as a carpenter led to the collapsed vertebrae.

In reviewing his documentation, I noticed the name of Dr. Carillo M.D. Dr. Carillo practiced on the Mexican side of the Texas border and was well known for inappropriate and heavy use of cortisone preparations. The patient had gone to Dr. Carillo for "generalized aches and pains"; diagnosed by Dr. Carillo as "arthritis". He felt 100 percent better on the medication prescribed by the Mexican physician. Dr. Carillo assured him the medications did not contain steroids (cortisone) of any kind. The patient/claimant gave us samples of the assorted colored pills he got from Dr. Carillo. They all contained significant amounts of cortisone and he, in effect, had been taking massive daily doses. This was unquestionably what caused his vertebrae to collapse. The case was dismissed as non-work related.

It's difficult enough sorting out the credentials and abilities of health care providers in this country. Why look for trouble outside the United States?

Chiropractors (DC); some people swear by them, and interestingly, not enough swear at them. Unmistakable harm by inappropriate treatment and/or faulty diagnoses goes unchallenged. Some of it has to do with whose paying the bills, good *listening* skills, denial and placebo effect. Their ads pretty much parallel the

Oriental Medicine ads: preposterous claims for every medical condition known to man.

A guard at the Test Site sought my opinion three weeks after experiencing a forward fall, landing on his outstretched hand. His contract allowed him to see whomever he chose, for work related injuries. He went to a Chiropractor for pain in his wrist and elbow. The Chiropractor took his own x-rays: chest, shoulder views and multiple extremity views. The Chiropractor's diagnosis was strain/sprain and his treatment was daily heat and manipulation. The elbow pain got worse so the man decided to get my opinion.

I had him bring in the Chiropractor's x-rays. Most were unnecessary…like the chest x-ray and shoulder views. The other x-rays were of poor quality (under or over developed and not in focus), improperly labeled with inappropriate views (positioning of the part being x-rayed). Those were the expert opinions of a Board Certified MD radiologist.

In addition, the Chiropractor did not recognize the fracture of the head of the radius, which one of his x-rays did manage to show. Obviously, applying heat and daily manipulation was not appropriate fracture treatment. I offered to testify (at no charge) if the guard would sue for malpractice. He refused. I advised his employer to deny payment to the Chiropractor. They ignored my recommendation. The Chiropractor got paid and continues to take worthless, inappropriate x-rays; make unsubstantiated diagnoses; sell health supplements....and all the rest. I can assure you, if the guard had been personally liable for the bill, the course of events would have been different. His elbow healed with my treatment and follow-up physical therapy. He saw the Chiropractic visits as only being an *inconvenience; i.e.* he had no out-of-pocket expenses and got full pay for limited duty.

Contrast that to the following case during my family practice years in Peekskill, N.Y. (1960's). That case did suffer permanent damage.

It was Saturday morning, 1967. I was up to my ears with patients waiting to be seen during my morning, walk-in, office hours. In those days, I was available 24/7 and I made house calls. I always took emergencies first, but everything else was first come, first served. The local hospital had no such thing as an emergency room staff. I answered the hospital's call for help as required. Many cases were sent directly to my office.

A new patient was wheel-chaired in by her husband on that busy Saturday morning. I asked if she needed immediate care. She told me she could wait. I looked around and told her it might be two hours. She smiled and said, " that will be fine." She turned out to be my last patient of morning—by then it was 1:45 PM.

She had been working around the house several weeks earlier and developed acute low back pain. It had come on suddenly and radiated to her left buttock and leg. She tried liniment rubs, heating pad, a tight girdle and various over the counter pain pills. She was forced to stay in bed because of the pain. She noticed it got worse if she had to cough. She was most comfortable lying on her side with her knees bent and the hips slightly flexed.

A typical family practitioner (MD) in 1967 would have diagnosed her condition as a sciatic nerve impingement due to a bulging or ruptured disc… until proven otherwise. She would have been hospitalized with a complete history and medical exam (special attention to neurologic signs and symptoms), appropriate x-rays (MRI's, CAT scans and ultrasound hadn't been invented yet), and a neurosurgeon or orthopedist asked to consult. The specialist might have ordered a myelogram, which is no longer used.

Unfortunately, she went to a Chiropractor. He took a "bunch of x-rays" and told her she had a bad case of *lumbago* (not an accepted medical term). He applied ultrasound to the back, sold her a cumbersome metal corset, sold her three different herbal medications and advised she would need to see him daily for about three weeks. She noticed numbness and tingling (pins and needles) in both lower extremities during the first week of Chiropractic massage and manipulation. The Chiropractor applied more aggressive manipulation the second week, which led to complete rupture of the bulging disc, and acute paraplegia. I referred her to a hospital in lower Westchester County. They operated to relieve pressure on the compromised nerves but she never regained full function of her legs. She waddled like a duck when she walked.

We didn't have computers with Google search engines in those days.

I asked a medical librarian to search the literature for me….the old fashioned way…very labor intensive. I showed my patient articles where others had been made paraplegic and quadriplegic through faulty diagnoses and inappropriate treatments by Chiropractors. I told her she had an airtight legal case for malpractice, and I showed her awards made for similar cases. She never sued, despite being permanently disabled, burdened with medical bills, and eventually divorced from her husband.

Taking advantage of a vulnerable person is certainly not limited to Chiropractors. Sadly, it's a recurring universal trait, manifest in all human interactions. However, giving legitimacy to this type of health care provider, in my opinion, compounds the insult and is egregious beyond words.

Look at the Yellow Pages in your phone book. Chiropractors target audiences similar to those of Oriental Medicine, Faith healers and other non-allopathic entrepreneurs. They love people with pain symptoms and third party insurance coverage, like worker's comp, auto accidents or Medicare. The patient is free of significant financial responsibility. This diminishes and/or eliminates patient motivation to shop wisely and critically review the billing. The insurance payer has limited control of the service provider. I've seen case after case where the insurer complains of endless visits and tests, but is powerless to curtail the runaway provider.

Another group of patients vulnerable to *alternative health care providers*, are those with functional complaints, as opposed to physical problems like tumors, trauma or infections. People with fatigue, digestive complaints, headaches and myalgias. They are suffering and their symptoms and discomforts are real. Serious, treatable causes must always be ruled out. Allopathic physicians (MD's), in general, do a poor job with these patients, if they can't find an organic or physical cause. They often refer to them as *crocks, hypochondriacs,* or just plain *nuts*. Those types of patients take a lot of time, are not easily helped and may never be cured. Those patients are too often abandoned by qualified doctors and left to drift into the clutches of entrepreneurs and charlatans. They become desperate and fail to heed the caveat of CONSUMER BEWARE.

I received a Chiropractic flier in the mail. What's your reaction? To me it sounds more like an ad for a Las Vegas-style buffet.

WHAT DO YOU WANT FOR CHRISTMAS?
- *LIFE WITHOUT PAIN?*
- *MORE ENERGY?*
- *BETTER HEALTH?*

WE CAN HELP (APPROXIMATE TOTAL VALUE $255)
FREE INITIAL EXAM
FREE X-RAYS (as necessary)
WHY FREE?
BECAUSE OUR GIFT TO YOU IS TO SHOW YOU HOW CHIROPRACTIC CAN HELP YOU.
IT COULD CHANGE YOUR LIFE.
(MUST PRESENT FLIER — NEW PATIENTS ONLY)

An Associated Press release in June 2005, stated that the government, in 2001, paid chiropractors close to 285 million in services that should not have been billed to Medicare. The government maintained it should not have paid for maintenance manipulations. Rather, it should only have paid for, "manipulations designed to improve". How long do you think it took chiropractors to adjust the wording? Gaming the system exists among all health care providers. My point here is to exclude chiropractors (and oriental medicine) from billing in the first place. I'll address Medicare, Medicaid and other insurance fraud and abuse in the chapter on hospitals and institutions.

For general information on Podiatry (DPM) try interamericanmed.net.

"There are currently 8 colleges of podiatric medicine in the United States (2007). Successful completion of one of these programs leads to a Doctor of Podiatric Medicine (DPM) degree. Many of these programs are affiliated and either partially or fully integrated with an MD or DO school.

The education consists of 2 years of basic science/general medicine courses followed by two years of clinical rotations, similar to regular medical school. These rotations are done in non-hospital-based clinics as well as major hospitals and deal with general medicine, basic podiatric medicine, and podiatric surgery. Research opportunities for medical students are available during these four years.

DPM students take the NBPME (National Board of Podiatric Medical Examiner's) and match for Podiatric Medicine and Surgery (PM&S) residences, 2–3 years long. Podiatrists may practice in all of the US and are licensed by each states independent Podiatric Board."

Podiatrists knowledge and training for care of the foot and ankle is just as good as any MD orthopedist (their major competitors), and generally better than most other physicians, regardless of what letters append their names. Many take their own x-rays and do surgery in their office clinics. Hospitals can give them medical and surgical privileges limited to the foot and ankle.

Pressures arise in all disciplines of legitimate health care providers, and podiatrists are definitely included. I've coined a word for southern Nevada physicians who succumb to the national disease of greed and ego: I call it *Vegatization*. You may have a different name for it, but it's globally ubiquitous. The fact remains that delivering health care by the rules is like walking a tightrope. Office overheads, malpractice premiums, required worker health plans, unrealistic fee re-embursements and fierce competition tempt practitioners to game the system. If the practitioner has dominant greed and ego "genes", there are no limits to the game…as they see it.

If you look in the Yellow Pages, you'll see the legitimate spectrum of podiatric care. They've been well trained to take care of: bunions and hammer toes, ingrown and deformed nails, corns, calluses and warts, diabetic foot care, arthritic foot conditions, skins disorders, foot and ankle sports medicine/injuries, foot and ankle trauma, physical therapy, heel problems, arch pain and spurs, orthotics, and fungus. They are licensed to write for prescription medications.

After years of expense and training, they are allowed to practice within a limited anatomic field (ankle and foot), competing with MD's, DO's, Chiropractors, orthotic technicians and self proclaimed foot and ankle aficionados. In my opinion, they have not been afforded the respect they deserve from MD and DO's, and they usually do not generate the fees given MD orthopedists, dermatologists and internists rendering the same type and quality care to the foot and ankle. It's no wonder some podiatrists turn to the practice of over x-raying in the office, run unnecessary laboratory tests, sell medications, inflate the number of office visits or do ill-advised surgeries. The latest money deal has been the sale of *custom* orthotics. The profit margins are huge. We used to be content with getting a Dr. Scholl's shoe insert…Medicare and other re-embursements have turned it into a booming industry. Understanding the dynamics does not excuse illegal or unethical behavior by any health care provider. However, understanding should stimulate thought toward improvement and correction within the system.

I would like to see Podiatry licensed by a combined MD/DO state licensing board, and this is an example for my bias.

There were two podiatrists in Las Vegas who, in the 80's, were doing bunionectomies in numbers suggesting a regional epidemic. One of their cases came to my attention as Medical Director for the Nevada Test Site.

A 20-year old man tried to return to work 6 weeks after bunionectomies on both feet. He had gone to the podiatrists because of pain in his feet. They had diagnosed bilateral bunions as the cause of his foot pain and they showed him their x-rays as part of their pitch for surgery. A bunionectomy at this age is not common, let alone bilaterally. Return to work was out of the question due to persistent swollen, red operative sites. The surgeries had been performed in their own outpatient facilities. I sent over the patient's signed release for medical records, operative records and x-rays. They were not forthcoming.

I registered a complaint with the Nevada Board of Podiatry. Turns out I was just one of a long list of complaints. The Board of Podiatry never answered me and the podiatrists never gave me the records. I advised the patient to supoena the records and file a malpractice suit. He failed to do either.

The local newspaper eventually reported that the Nevada Podiatric Board, acting on numerous complaints, issued a temporary license suspension and a fine. The two podiatrists were subsequently allowed to resume practice, which they did under a new office name. To me, the Podiatric Board's lack of appropriate action makes them as guilty of criminal activity as their podiatric members. It also casts a negative cloud over other well trained, ethical podiatrists. If the patient had wanted to pursue damages, he would have had to hire his own lawyer and go to court on his time and at his expense; not many can do that.

The caveat here, as with all non-emergency medical or surgical care, paraphrases what my carpenter father repeatedly told me: MEASURE TWO OR THREE TIMES, BEFORE YOU CUT ONCE. Obtain second or third opinions, research your options on line or the old fashioned ways; talk to other patients who used the same health care provider. Be very clear about what is being said to you. Ask for a written copy of proposals, projected outcomes and risks. It's your responsibility to understand the realistic risks and benefits of your proposed care.

By now you should realize that words present different perceptions to different people. Those intent on misleading an intended target are masters at strategic omissions and /or deliberate misinformation. You've been given facts and case examples demonstrating why "all physicians/doctors are not created equal." What about other "doctors"?

There are many, many legitimate doctor/people. As with MD's and DO's, it's up to you to carefully look at what doctorate they claim, what school they attended (reputable and recognized or was it a mail-order mill?), what regulatory statues apply and how well are they enforced. There are doctorates in pharmacy, psychology, bioengineering, anatomy and physiology, chemistry and physics…to name a few in the science fields. Specialized doctorates hold critical teaching positions in our 4-year medical schools, especially in the first two years. When seeking medical help, you need to be knowledgeable about the credentials and limitations of your caregiver. Make sure they're suited for the service you seek and need. Do you know detailed differences between:

    An intern versus an internist?
    A resident versus an attending?
    A psychologist versus a psychiatrist?
    An optometrist versus an ophthalmologist?
    A neurologist versus a neurosurgeon?
    A physiatrist versus a physical therapist?
    A geneticist versus a genealogist?
    A medical examiner versus a coroner?

Then you also need to know the many categories of physician extenders…and their rapidly changing authority and responsibilities:

- Nurse practitioner (NP)
- Licensed practical nurse (LPN)
- Physician assistant (PA)
- Licensed/certified technicians (laboratory, radiology, etc.)
- Registered Nurse (RN)

If you, or a friend have computer access, you can easily determine who you're actually dealing with. Take the time to investigate. The odds are not in your favor if you neglect your obligations and just "roll the dice and hope for the best."

SavvySenior.org had a very good article on "how to give your doctor a checkup." I give you the recommendations with the author's, Jim Miller's, permission:

"FINDING DR. RIGHT

The Internet has become the single greatest source for locating and evaluating physicians. Whether you're researching a new doctor or looking to learn more about your current doctor(s), there are several online resources that provide basic data on just about every licensed doctor in the United States. Here are some good ones to help you get started.

- **Vitals.com:** a free Web resource (www.vitals.com) that will help you find, evaluate and choose a doctor based on his or her training, expertise, consumer ratings and recommendations from other doctors. You can also rate doctors and leave comments for other to see. Other sites to check that offer similar services include www.ratemds.com , www.findadoc.com, www.careseek.com,

www.thehealthcarescoop.com and www.drscore.com.
- **American Medical Association:** offers a DoctorFinder service(webapps.ama-assn.org/doctor-finder) that provides free information on virtually every licensed physician in the United States, including their educational history, medical specialties and hospital admitting privileges.

DOCTOR'S CHECKUP

After you find a few doctors you're interested in, here are some additional sources that can help you dig a little deeper. To check into your doctor's board certification status, for example, visit the American Board of Medical Specialties www.abms.org or call (866) 275-2267. And to learn about any disciplinary actions taken against doctors, your state medical licensing board probably is your best resource (remember that this chapter warns you of problems with different "types" of physicians and their separate licensing boards…this article deals mainly with allopathic (MD) physicians.) The Federation of State Medical Boards Web site has direct links to every state board at www.fsmb.org/directory_smb.html where you can search for free. Or you can go to www.docinfo.org and request a physician profile (for $10) that includes license and disciplinary status.

If you're looking for more information, there are several fee-based services that can help, including Health Grades (www.healthgrades.com) which provides reports ($29.95 each) that cover education and training, board certification, professional misconduct or disciplinary action and satisfaction scores from patients. Consumer's Checkbook (www.checkbook.org) is another neat service that can help you search for top-rated doctors that have actually been recommended by other doctors. Its database lists 20,000 physicians, in 30 different fields of specialty, in 50 metro areas. They charge $24.95 for a two-year subscription.

WHAT TO KNOW

Once you have found a few names of doctors you might want to try, here are some additional things you need to find out, which you can easily do by calling their offices.

- Are they accepting new patients?
- Do they accept your specific health insurance plan? You also can find this out by visiting your health plan's Web site. To search for doctors that accept Medicare go to www.medicare.gov/physician, or call (800) 633-4227.

- **Where is their clinic or office located? Is it easy for you to get there?**
- **What are the office hours?**
- **How long does it take to get an appointment?**
- **Does the doctor have a relationship with the hospital you prefer?**
- **Is the doctor available after hours or on weekends?**
- **Does the doctor (or a nurse or physician assistant) give advice over the phone or via e-mail for common medical problems?**
- **If the doctor is of foreign decent does he/she speak clear, understandable English?"**

Savvy Senior, P.O. Box 5443, Norman, OK 73070, or www.savvysenior.org.

If the patient has a medical problem and /or language-culture problem, he/she will need appropriate help in finding and communicating with the healthcare provider.

CHAPTER II

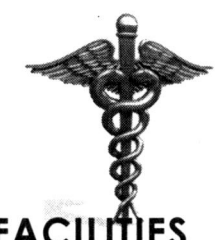

HOSPITALS AND OUTPATIENT FACILITIES

Times have changed. The echo-boomers and millennial generation live by the computer, worship the art of marketing and seek to turn everything into a commercial enterprise. Around the world money talks; in Las Vegas it sings. Here's an example of Las Vegas' pioneering entrepreneurial spirit:

Sunrise Hospital (HCA—Hospital Corporation of America) was probably the first in the country to provide valet parking service for patients and/or guests (1960's). Parking attendants wore quasi cowboy or cowgirl attire…..or in warm weather, cocktail waitress inspirations for women; i.e. lot's of cleavage with visible, bouncing buns. Over the years it has taken care of entertainment celebrities, royalty, visitors and locals. The hospital likes to drop names like tennis star, Andre Agassi, being born there, or Elvis Presley being treated there.

Sunrise Hospital has had many positive firsts for southern Nevada, like the first neonatal unit in the state and partnering with University Medical Center (not-for-profit teaching hospital) to help fund and teach medical students and postgraduate students in pediatric settings at the University of Nevada School of Medicine. They've also tried monetary incentives worthy of discussion at the Wharton School of Business.

Mr. David Brandsness, a very capable hospital administrator, wanted to boost weekend hospital occupancy. He offered a cash incentive as well as drawings for cruises, if patients would check in on Fridays. Very little elective activity takes place during hospital weekends. Insurance companies were not happy with the practice. They accurately pointed out that it was their money that covered the largely unnecessary hospital days. No harm trying......or was there?

Peekskill, New York, in the 1960's, had one community hospital serving a population of approximately 200,000. Blue Shield/Blue Cross was the major health insurer and the hospital accepted most plans as full payment. Physicians and their families were given significant hospital and provider courtesy when it came to billing. Most rural physicians extended courtesy to colleagues, their families, allied health professionals and clergy.

Medicare emerged in the late 60's and it covered most qualified hospital stays, with insignificant co-pays. The post World War II years, late 40's to the early 70's, was considered by most physicians to be the GOLDEN YEARS OF MEDICAL PRACTICE: we enjoyed minimal bureaucratic intrusion and hassle, with liberal reembursements. Imagine my shock when I came to Las Vegas in July 1973.

We had 8 hospitals in southern Nevada for a population of 250,000: one County run, not-for-profit teaching hospital; one not-for-profit hospital started in 1947 by seven Adrian Dominican sisters from Michigan; 3 major privately run hospitals; 2 smaller privately run hospitals and one privately run women's specialty hospital. Blue Cross/Blue Shield had a miniscule piece of the market and courtesy consideration from hospitals or providers was extremely rare. The hospitals set their rates, took patient insurance and expected the patient to make up the difference.

Both Las Vegas newspapers reported Las Vegas sixth in the nation for hospital markups (September 10, 2004). The national markup average was 232 percent while Nevada's <u>average</u> was 276 percent. This means the hospital billed $276 for every $100 service cost. The highest markup in Las Vegas was 526 percent. Interestingly to me, the hospital with the highest markup was the least desirable… cost does not necessarily reflect value. The for-profit hospitals ran between 400 to 500 percent markups. These numbers do not reflect other creative billing practices like cost shifting, owning medical supply companies so you could sell to yourself, and unbundling laboratory, diagnostic and service charges.

<u>PROTECTIVE MEASURES---WHAT YOU NEED TO KNOW AND DO</u>

- **Have a family doctor and get in writing what that doctor provides with respect to office hours, after hour coverage, hospital coverage and insurance coverage; i.e. does he or she provide hospital care or will you be placed into the care of a *hospital intensivist*?**
- **Get in writing, what your insurance plan covers and what your co-payments will be. Have a <u>written</u> understanding that you only want health care providers who accept Medicare, Medicaid and/or your other insurance plans. Compliance may be impossible in an emergency situation, but your healthcare provider will have to justify an alleged emergency should questions arise.**
- <u>**NEVER PAY OUT OF POCKET---UNTIL YOUR INSURDED PORTION HAS BEEN FULLY PAID.**</u> **If you pay your co-insurance and /or whatever incidental charges are added,**

and it's later determined you paid too much, you most assuredly will have a very hard time getting re-embursed.
- It's your responsibility to review all bills for accuracy, and to report disputes to the proper regulatory bodies, if you can't reach a resolution with the hospital and/or providers.

Here's a personal example of what needs to be done with contested billing.

My wife and I stopped to visit a physician friend for a few days in Boynton Beach, Florida, prior to starting a Caribbean cruise. My wife slipped in the shower and got a deep cut on the front of her ankle. It was around 11:00 PM. The only place for medical care was the emergency room of a small area hospital. We checked in, provided our Medicare and co-insurance information. We were told the hospital and treating physician accepted our insurance and would follow required processing protocols. The place did not appear that busy, but it did take two hours to be seen and another hour to be treated. I was not happy with the cursory examination of the wound, or the cavalier attitude toward maintaining a sterile environment. The ankle did become swollen and red within 24 hours. We were on our way to boarding our cruise ship which prevented a return to the treating hospital. I put my wife on antibiotics and removed two metal clips to allow infected wound drainage. It took several weeks to completely heal. The final result was acceptable, even though the emergency medical care was open to criticism.

    I received a non-itemized bill from the hospital for $980 (physician and hospital services). I reminded them that they accepted Medicare and secondary insurance, and that my secondary insurer guaranteed usual and customary fees for emergency care. I asked that the bill be submitted to those two carriers, and that they itemize services, as required in all billings. It took two years to resolve the alleged debt. I repeatedly contacted the Florida fiscal intermediary for Medicare. I contacted the Attorney General's office in the state of Georgia (where the hospital had contracted with a bill-collecting firm). I insisted on itemization of the bill. I informed them of the postcare infection and I refused to pay anything until the insurance coverage was properly resolved. I kept copies of all correspondence. The resolution provided the hospital with $97.00 for the entire service (paid by Medicare). I can guarantee that, had I paid anything along the way, it would never have been returned. If you know (or think) the billing is not accurate, notify the provider. If still not satisfied, notify the insurer and a medical ombudsman (patient advocate) in your city, county or state beauracracy. Don't pay out of pocket until you're satisfied the charges are correct and your insurance has paid its obligations.

Here's a Las Vegas case in which the hospital responded promptly and properly, but the physician and regulating agencies did not.

My neighbor's 34-year old daughter, single and between jobs, twisted her ankle causing a trimalleolar fracture; i.e. fractures of all three stabilizing bones of the ankle. Everyone knows trauma leads to bleeding and swelling. This makes it important to operate as soon as possible…before the area swells and/or circulation is compromised. The patient was properly diagnosed and cared for at a Quick Care facility operated by the teaching hospital. She was sent to the teaching hospital, by ambulance, within one hour of diagnosis and stabilization.

She had no insurance due to leaving her last employment and still in the process of being accepted in a new job as a court stenographer. She was assigned to the orthopedist on call and seen by a DO orthopedic fellow. The DO was a fourth year DO medical student from Michigan who, in effect, was hired by local orthopedists to see hospital patients assigned to the service; i.e. having no doctor of their own. The so-called *fellowship* was not accredited; it was a convenience for attending orthopedists. They used the so-called fellow to avoid coming to the hospital at inconvenient hours. The so-called *Fellowship* had no formal, written set of teaching responsibilities, quality control, oversight or meaningful certification. The attending orthopedist on call was obligated, by contract, to see an acute injury within 30 minutes of being called. He got $4500 a day for being on call…whether he was needed or not….and he could bill insurers, if the patient was insured. This patient was given inappropriate, unsupervised care by the *DO fellow*, and was not seen by the attending for 48 hours. The attending operated on the third day. The hospital bill was $13,000. The orthopedist's bill was $5,000. The orthopedist failed to inform the patient she was entitled to free follow-up care in the hospital's outpatient clinic. Instead, he had her come to his office where he repeatedly took unnecessary x-rays and added follow-up charges.

My neighbor asked if I could do anything about the bills. I reviewed all the records and called the hospital. I pointed out the hospital's liability in allowing an unsupervised *fellow* to inappropriately render medical care, having a contract orthopedist violate the terms of his contract, placing a patient in danger and causing unnecessary hospital days and service charges. They reduced the hospital bill to $3000 and worked out a mutually acceptable payment schedule.

I did not fair as well with the orthopedist. I quickly discovered that well-trained did not translate to well-balanced. He would not talk to me, or answer my letters. I advised the patient to stop seeing him. She was healing well and did not need unnecessary visits, x-rays and more charges. She was reluctant to go to court, even though I offered to testify at no charge. She still would need to hire a lawyer. She did follow my advice to not pay any more money to the orthopedist. I wrote letters to the hospital executive committee, the State Board of Medical Examiners, the State Ombudsman and the Joint Commission for Hospital Accreditation. No official action was taken, but the orthopedist did stop sending bills to the patient.

How are hospitals supposed to work? How are credentials verified, privileges granted and quality of care overseen? Here is a description of the intended process.

The business side of the hospital is the administrative staff. The hospital administrator is selected by the hospital's board of directors and he/she may be an MD or DO physician with business and administrative skills. Generally, the administrator is not a medically trained person. The medical staff comes under a hospital medical director and/or chief of staff. A medical director is hired by the administrator. The chief of staff is elected by the medical staff. The administrator has the final word in policy, funding and oversight.

Applicants for hospital privileges are screened by the Chief of Staff's office. Hospitals write the rules for staff priviledges. A medical degree does not guarantee hospital priviledges. The chief of staff's secretarial pool makes sure information on applications for hospital privileges is accurate: i.e. approved training programs, board certifications, state licensure and no past legal violations. Bad apples do slip through; as a result of deliberate false statements and/or procedural errors. The chief of staff chairs the executive committee, composed of heads of the various hospital departments (surgery, medicine, pediatrics, obstetrics/gynecology, etc.)

New medical staff approvals are usually assigned an attending to oversee and evaluate actual performance during a probationary period. For example, a staff neurosurgeon will assist or observe the new kid on the block. If there's a problem, it would be promptly brought to the chief's attention. In my opinion, teaching hospitals generally run a tighter ship; i.e. more people looking over each other's shoulders. However, there are no guarantees that monitoring physicians will follow through with his/her due diligence.

With this organizational understanding, you, as a patient may file a complaint or seek an explanation from the hospital's administrator, medical director and/or chief of staff. If these entities do not satisfactorily handle the matter, then you need to contact appropriate city, county, state and federal health-regulating agencies.

Huge problems can arise with regulating agencies, as was demonstrated in southern Nevada, March 2008. Two cases of Hepatitis C caught the attention of the Clark County Health Department. It was quickly determined that a private gastroenterology practice was putting patients at risk with unacceptable re-use of syringes and multiple dose anesthesia vials. There were other alleged violations relating to colonoscopy examinations. Bottom line; over 50,000 patients had to be notified, the federal Centers for Disease Control and Prevention (CDC) was called in and at least 9 confirmed cases of Hepatitis C were traced to the endoscopy practice with a hundred additional cases probably related to that group's practice. The Nevada Board of Medical Examiners, The Clark County Health Department and the State Health Agency did nothing to immediately close the clinic and suspend licenses. It took the Mayor of Las Vegas and the City Council to halt operations at the clinic, by yanking their business license. I won't go into the sordid details of political corruption and medical malpractice…not to mention the devastating effects on patient lives. To top it off, little has been done (in my informed opinion) to punish the perpetrators or to ensure corrective action. To paraphrase something Thomas Jefferson once said about democracy: continual vigilance (and collective resolve) is necessary to ensure intended function and survival. The finger points in all directions.

What about hospital outpatient clinics, or privately run clinics? Hospital outpatient care was originally touted as a way to save money without compromising quality of care. In my opinion, it hasn't panned out. Outpatient surgical care still appears as expensive as inpatient care, and in some instances not medically acceptable. For example, I cringe when a patient is sent home, *by the clock*, still groggy from anesthesia, with cavalier lip service cautioning the patient about bleeding, pain, infection, falling or other trauma.

The hospitals make more money with short stays and outpatient care because insurance coverage often pays a set amount for a given diagnosis or procedure. If the hospital can do it in less than the allotted time, using less of everything else, it obviously generates a bigger profit margin.

The same holds true for privately run specialty hospitals, outpatient surgeries and clinics. Privately run entities face less operational scrutiny (like the podiatrists described in the previous chapter). Cash up front operations are notorious for ignoring or bending rules and regulations of accepted medical practices: examples: methadone clinics, liposuction, cosmetic centers, weight reduction surgical clinics and medical diet programs, antiaging centers and countless schemes for *alternative* health care. Many follow the rules but sadly, too many of these activities do not get light shined on them until tragedy strikes. It comes down to BUYER BEWARE; IF IT SOUNDS TOO GOOD TO BE TRUE, IT PROBABLY ISN'T TRUE.

Nursing home and extended care facilities: they all have mandates and regulations but oversight is problematic due to skimpy funding, lack of legislative will, inspector understaffing and perfunctory penalties.

Money plays a big part in what the patient receives for institutional care. The average nursing type facility runs between $2000 and $3000 a month for a room, meals and minimal additional care. Additional costs, like doctor visits, nursing supervision and laboratory tests, may add substantially to the monthly bill. The patient and/or the family need to carefully screen for the availability of their specific needs, and they need to keep a critical eye on the quality of services once they select a facility.

No chapter on institutional care would be complete without mention of HOSPICE. The concept started in England and the first United States hospice was established in Connecticut. The second hospice in this country and the first west of the Mississippi, is the Nate Adelson Hospice in Las Vegas, Nevada. To those who think Las Vegas is a parasitic, hedonistic creation for man's pursuit of instant pleasure, I invite them to visit this beautiful setting in the heart of the valley, next to the western edge of the campus of the University of Nevada Las Vegas. It's creators, staff and mission are tributes to man's highest moral and spiritual commitments for fellow human beings.

Hospice philosophy and mission are stated in the following:

TO CURE SOMETIMES
TO RELIEVE OFTEN
TO COMFORT ALWAYS
(author unknown)

End of life is generally a forgotten part of medicine. America appears to be a death denying society. The public worships youth and beauty while the medical community sees death as a failure. Dr. Karen Cross MD, FAAHPM, Vice President of Physician Services (Adelson Hospice) stated:

"Hospice is a philosophy of care focusing on the relief of symptoms with an emphasis on quality of life, not quantity of life. The goal is to keep the patient at home (or in the Hospice facility) with optimal control of pain, physical symptoms, psychological, social and spiritual problems. This is accomplished through an interdisciplinary team approach."

Many families are reluctant to ask for help and/or consider admission to any type of care facility. They view it in terms of guilt relative to implied obligations. Terminally ill patients, however, are frequently best served by hospice care; in or out of the home. No one is turned away because of money, and individualized strategies are the goal, not the exception. Don't feel guilty if you or your loved ones are faced with end of life medical care decisions.

The nation has a long way to go in understanding, accepting and utilizing hospice-type care. It's important to spouses, children and friends---as well as the patient. If your healthcare provider is reluctant to learn about it, then it's up to you to get the facts. The founding woman in England, Dame Cicely Saunders, St. Christopher 's Hospice, London summed it up:

"YOU MATTER BECAUSE OF WHO YOU ARE. YOU MATTER UNTIL THE LAST MOMENT OF YOUR LIFE, AND WE WILL DO ALL WE CAN NOT ONLY TO HELP YOU DIE PEACEFULLY, BUT ALSO TO LIVE UNTIL YOU DIE."

If you don't know where to start, ask the social service department of your local hospital for recommendations, and visit available facilities.

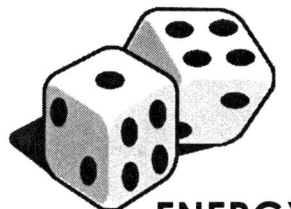 # CHAPTER III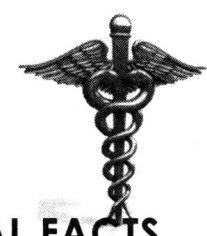

ENERGY NEEDS AND MEDICAL FACTS

Understanding elementary facts of generating energy from nuclear sources (as well as other alternatives), and understanding medical implications is vital to intelligent and necessary decisions for our country's energy independence, and the world's well being.

The Las Vegas Review Journal, May 1, 2005, reprinted a special to the Washington Post entitled, THE KEY TO OUR ENERGY FUTURE. The sentinel message read : "clean energy is impossible without global expansion of nuclear power." The article was written by John Rich, Director General of the World Nuclear Association, and former U.S. Ambassador to the International Atomic Energy Agency and other UN agencies in Vienna, from 1993-2001. He went on to say:

"Every authoritative energy analysis points to an inescapable imperative: humankind cannot conceivably achieve a global clean-energy revolution without a rapid expansion of nuclear power to generate electricity, produce hydrogen for tomorrow's vehicles and drive seawater desalination plants to meet a fast-emerging world water crises.

Today (2005) some 440 civil nuclear reactors, in 30 countries, comprising 2/3 of humankind, produce 16 percent of the world's electricity. Under current plans, these nations will construct several hundred more reactors by 2030. China and India will lead the way, but the expansion will be broad-based."

If current nuclear fusion projects prove successful, cheaper, cleaner, safer energy sources will be an added alternative to currently operating fission plants. The future can be exciting and productive.

I was Medical Director for Reynolds Electric and Engineering (Reeco) for 18 years (1973–1991). Reeco was the prime contractor to the Nevada Operations Office of the Department of Energy. I am well qualified to speak about nuclear subjects; bombs, energy generation, nuclear waste storage, transportation of partially spent fuel rods, terrorism threats, medical facts and political/economic realities.

FACTS ABOUT THE NEVADA TEST SITE (NTS)

Mercury, the main entrance to the 1400 square mile testing area, is approximately 65 miles north of Las Vegas, on Route 95. That land had been part of the Nellis Bombing and Gunnery Range prior to becoming the atomic testing area. Three laboratories; Lawrence Livermore. Sandia and Los Alamos worked with the Department of Energy (DOE) and Department of Defense (DOD) to verify reliability of existing nuclear weapons and to develop new systems. In the 18 years I was Medical Director, we had one minor radiation-related incident.

It was a Monday morning and a radiation monitor was teaching a class how to handle a small amount of a radioactive substance. The material was safely transported in a small lead container. The monitor's mind must have been on other matters as he opened the container, reached in and brought out the radioactive substance with his bare hand. He quickly realized what he had done and put the radioactive source back into the container and closed the lid. No students in the room received significant exposure. The analysis and handling of the event required a basic understanding of radiation physics and medicine.

- One has to know the properties of the radiation source; i.e. the type of radiation emitted; alpha, beta or gamma.

- One has to know the distance from the radiation source and the length of *exposure* (versus *contamination*; internal and/or external).
- One has to take into account the presence of shielding.
- One has to know basic medical facts to monitor for acute, intermediate and long term biologic responses, as well as treatment options.

This case was easy to analyze. We knew the radiation source, the distance from the source and exposure time. We quickly calculated the radiation dose received to the hand and forearm; the rest of the monitor's body did not receive significant exposure. However, we did look at blood samples for systemic (general) radiation effects as well as carefully inspecting the hand and forearm. The monitor showed no measurable response; not even a reddening of the hand or forearm. This serves to illustrate the wide margin of safety between allowable radiation exposures and dosages causing measurable adverse medical effects. It also explains why we can live comfortably with normal daily background radiation; i.e. flying coast to coast, for example, gives us a radiation dose equivalent to one chest x-ray.

This was the only radiation incident in the 18 years I was medical director for the Department of Energy's Nevada office for atomic testing.

Being anti-nuclear is generally considered a vote-getter in a state like Nevada. It is not necessarily true in the 15 counties outside of Washoe (Reno) and Clark (Las Vegas). Politicians pander to the public's desire for a risk free environment. They make ridiculous promises, promote unrealistic scenarios and disseminate deliberate misinformation.

Here are a few basic facts about nuclear generation of energy:

1. **Nuclear generation is approximately 50 years old, readily available, safe, inexpensive and clean. Coal-fired plants put out radioactive effluent (polonium 210) and carbon waste; nuclear generating plants do not.**
2. **Nuclear power plants can provide electricity at 50 to 80 percent less cost than fossil fuel plants.**
3. **Unmatched safety record. There has never been a single radiation injury or death associated with commercial nuclear energy generation in the United States….. NOT ONE!**

4. Using natural gas to generate electrical energy is an egregious misuse of a natural resource. It should be used for home heating and cooking.
5. If France can produce over 80 percent of it's electricity from nuclear, and also use recycling, why have we been stagnant at 20 percent for over 30 years? Japan is also in the 70 percent range, and growing.
6. Three Mile Island was an engineering mishap. The safety measures worked. No one was harmed by radiation. In contrast, Russia was warned not to build a graphite reactor with no containment. Chernobyl was predictable and expected.
7. The anti-nuclear people like to state, "no level of radiation is safe". If you believe that, you'd better enter a lead cocoon the minute you're born, since we receive daily exposures from our ambient environment. Fortunately for us, there is a very wide margin of safety. That very margin of safety allows us to use radiation technology to diagnose and treat human beings.
8. 2004, China and India have ordered at least 20 reactors each for the next 10 years.
9. Read the book, A BRIGHTER TOMORROW, by Senator Pete Domenici (New Mexico).

Let's look at the practice of medicine and radiation. Doctors in general know very little about radiation medicine, unless they specialize in radiology and/or radiotherapy, or the specialty of Occupational and Environmental Medicine. Ask your family doctor (if you have one) if he or she can define terms like RAD, REM or GRAY? Do they know the acute symptoms of significant radiation exposure? Do they even know what numbers constitute significant exposure, i.e. the LD50? Do they know the difference between exposure and contamination?

All of this became extra important after 9/11…for obvious reasons. Unfortunately, little if any progress has been made in educating the professional and non-professional world. There have been deliberate omissions and strategic misinformation….the modus operandi of biased, special interests.

Take, for example, exposing food to ionizing radiation. It is an absolute scientific fact that exposing any type of food to ionizing radiation kills bacteria and viruses, and extends the shelf life of that food….WITHOUT ADVERSELY HARMING THE FOOD FOR HUMAN CONSUMPTION. The food does not become radioactive; it does not become toxic; it is perfectly safe. Congress, in all its wisdom, realized it could not change the erroneous mindset of the general public so it passed legislation using different terminology: it okayed "electronic pasteurization" of food (another term for irradiation). If we mandated that all meat, poultry, fish and vegetables be *"electronically pasteurized"*, we would never have to worry about E. Coli, Salmonella, Shigella, and all the other microbial hazards in the food chain. These are basic scientific facts. I fault our federal government, its institutions and elected officials, for failing to properly educate the public about irrefutable scientific facts.

The media needs to fess up to its misuse of power. Consider the following:

Las Vegas was very fortunate in having a physician by the name of Dr. Thorne Butler M.D. Dr. Butler was a founding partner of Associated Pathologists, a leading clinical laboratory in southern Nevada. He was internationally recognized as an eminent authority in forensic toxicology and laboratory medicine. You'd think that maybe this would make him an arrogant nerd. To the contrary, he was an avid outdoor enthusiast, quiet, humble, scrupulously honest with no limits to his community service. He was universally respected by the scientific world and well liked by his peers. He was appointed to the Nevada Department of Public Health by Governor Paul Laxalt in 1969, and was reappointed to 4-year terms until 1981. He was chairman of the State Department of Health from 1977 to 1981. Why wasn't he reappointed in 1981?

There was a private company handling disposal of very low level nuclear waste at Beatty, Nevada, about 100 miles north of Las Vegas. Some questions arose concerning the company's waste management practices vis-à-vis health and safety of the adjacent community and environment. Dr. Butler, as chairman of the State Health Department, was asked by the governor and one particular newspaper owner, to shut the company down. He gathered books, journals, and reports that literally stood two feet high....I'm not exaggerating. He read them all.

Since I was Board Certified in Occupational and Environmental Medicine (the second at the time so certified in the state of Nevada), and an expert in medical aspects of radiation medicine, Dr. Butler visited my office to discuss what he had researched. I asked him if he had really read all the material he carried in with him. He modestly said that he had scanned some and scrutinized the rest, but had critically reviewed it all.

I agreed with his conclusion that there was no justification to close the operation at

Beatty, Nevada. He refused to bow to unjustified pressure from the governor. A local newspaper carried the headline, "KILLERS AMONGST US". That newspaper deliberately and falsely accused Dr. Butler of endangering the lives of current and future generations of Nevadans by not closing the Beatty waste site. He was not reappointed to the state Department of Health in 1981. What a loss to the state, and what an injustice to a great human being. In my opinion, such unjust and dangerous *journalism* has increased as greed and special interests become more and more acceptable; i.e. WorldCom, Enron, HealthSouth, Abramoff, Cunningham of California, Stevens of Alaska, Wall Street, derivatives, subprime mortgages, Fannie Mae and Freddie Mac..... remember the movie WALL STREET, where Michael Douglas proclaimed, "GREED IS GOOD". We have become desensitized to evil; we have accepted normalization of deviant behavior.

Bottom line: we know how to effectively and safely handle ionizing radiation for the benefit of mankind. Let's educate the public to the facts and stop burying our heads in the sand.

A comment about solar, wind and geothermal sources of electrical energy. At best, these alternatives would only supply an estimated 5 to 10 percent of the nation's energy needs.

Let's add them to the mix of alternative energy sources but consider the following in terms of cost, efficiency and solving energy problems.

Nellis Air Force Base is the largest fighter base in the United States and is located in southern Nevada. A public relations man in Air Force uniform, appeared on local television, January 2008, to proudly announce the completion of a solar energy project at the air base. He said it would produce approximately 20 percent of the base's energy needs and save a million dollars a year (he also mentioned that was equivalent to the energy needs of approximately 13,000 homes). The project, he said, cost $100 million. Without factoring in ongoing operation and maintenance costs, it will take 100 years to write off the initial investment...your taxpayer dollars. The project used approximately 140 acres. Nevada alone has about 2 million people (2008). You do the math.

The Bush administration destabilized the agricultural industry by pushing ethanol production. For one thing we can buy ethanol cheaper from Brazil, than producing it ourselves. Secondly, we have foolishly pushed up the price of corn and everything connected to it in the food industry. Thirdly, the fuel industry has failed to provide easy access to stations with ethanol containing blends. Fourthly, producing ethanol takes lots of energy…more than we get from the ethanol end product and lastly, ethanol burns at about 65% of the power for an equal amount of gasoline. In other words, you pay less for ethanol blends at the pump and you get less mileage for the mixture.

Does it make sense to create an industry that destabilizes our food industry and comes out with a net loss of energy?

Hydrogen driven engines have been designed and could be put on the market. However, to cheaply produce hydrogen we need an inexpensive, clean energy source. Nuclear is the only current answer. Same goes for desalination of seawater, which is needed for many sections of the U.S. Have you driven over Hoover Dam lately? Lake Mead is below the critical level; over fifty percent down from its historical highs; the lowest level since it was completed in 1934.

We need an administration that will 'declare war' for energy solutions and create the equivalent of the Manhattan Project or NASA's race to the moon: define the goals, remove the red tape and obstructing special interests, fund the projects and let sound science prevail.

CHAPTER 1V

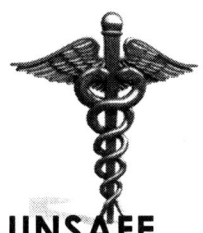

PARMACEUTICALS – SAFE OR UNSAFE

Data collection, accurate record keeping, quality control, integrity and timely review are basics for drug development. How good has the system been?

Pessimistic over-reactors like Dr. Sidney Wolfe and Dr. David Graham predict disastrous consequences without radical reform. It makes trial lawyers salivate, doomsayers jump for joy and provides grist for media hypesters. Dr. Sidney Wolfe is head of the Health Research Group of Public Citizen, an advocacy organization founded by Ralph Nader. Dr. David Graham is a Food and Drug Administration (FDA) researcher who testified before Congress in December 2004 with regard to Vioxx, Celebrex, Bextra and others.

Dr. Michael Crichton (physician/author) called for intelligent analysis in an article written for PARADE, December 5, 2004, entitled, LET'S STOP SCARING OURSELVES. He lists a string of dire predictions that never materialized. He stated: "human beings never tire of discussing the latest report that tells us the end is near."

- 1972 – The world was cooling and we were going to freeze to death.
- 2000 – Now the claim is the world is warming, creating new prospects for dying.
- 1960's to 70's – The world was going to starve to death because of overpopulation and famine. The birth rate did not explode as predicted, and food production is fine. Distribution is another story.
- A slew of unfounded health warnings: cancer from power lines, cell phones, saccharin, swine flu, cyclamates, endocrine disrupters, deodorants, electric razors, fluorescent lights, and computer terminals. Road rage as a sign of mental overload and killer bees dominating the Western Hemisphere—the list goes on.

Dr. Crichton summarized his point: "So many fears have turned out to be untrue or wildly exaggerated that I no longer get so excited about the latest one. Keeping fears in perspective leads me to ignore most of the frightening things I read and hear—or at least to take them with a pillar of salt.

For a time I wondered how it would feel without these fears and the frantic nagging concerns at the back of my mind. Actually, it feels just fine. I recommend it."

Being laid back has its merits, but burying one's head in the sand invites undesirable consequences. Embrace the positives and strive to correct the negatives. The patient does have a responsibility to proceed with caution, not panic and hysteria. Look at the facts. Discuss them with your doctor. Make sure you understand the risks versus benefits of your treatment options.

A prescription drug may take ten or more years of research and testing before receiving FDA approval. It's tested for safety, efficacy and comparative advantage to other medications being used for the same medical problem. The package insert for FDA approved medications carry detailed information on their biochemical properties, approved clinical indications, recommended dosage, possible side effects, drug interactions and contraindications. Off-label use of an approved medication is synonymous with experimental/not approved use…you and your doctor do it at your own risk. A physician would be wise to get written understanding from his patient before using anything off-label, and still understand he might be held liable for using the medication for non-sanctioned treatment.

Currently, the reporting system is mostly voluntary once a drug has passed FDA approval.

Physicians, pharmacists and patients are encouraged to report adverse reactions to the FDA and/or manufacturer. New findings will be added to the package insert, as warranted by reports from the field. If the risks outweigh the benefits, the FDA will require a *BLACKBOX WARNING* in the package insert; i.e. highlighting significant chances of serious side affects.

The FDA (law) has not required long term clinical follow-up once the drug went on the market. This means that the initial package insert only referred to studies reviewed by the FDA prior to allowing the drug onto the market.
Dr. Sidney Wolfe and Dr. David Graham take the position that if a drug is going to be used on a long term basis, the FDA should <u>require</u> long term follow-up studies by the manufacturer. Others claim this would be an unreasonable burden on the industry and would hinder pharmaceutical research and development. What would constitute an acceptable length of mandated follow-up study and how many patients would need to be included by such a mandate? No one has come up with hard numbers. 2007, however, saw legislation move in the direction of mandated follow-up of licensed medication. Evidence of intent in that direction is welcome but don't expect a rush to implementation.

Concerning Vioxx, and other COX-2 inhibitors like Celebrex and Bextra; these were a new group of *breakthrough* anti-inflammatory drugs offering pain relief with alleged minimal gastrointestinal irritation and/or bleeding. An alleged advantage over existing anti-inflammatory medications. When serious cardiovascular risks became evident, lawyers and their clients claimed negligence on the part of the FDA and pharmaceutical manufacturers for not issuing timely warnings and/or removing the product from the market. I believe there is blame all around: patients, physicians, FDA, manufacturers, lobbyists, legislators….everyone in the system; and as of January 2008, I don't see cooperation for meaningful reform. Special interests, conflicts of interest and no interests still prevail.

Consider the following:

1. Senator Chuck Grassley, R-Iowa, suggested during a Senate hearing that the FDA was too cozy with drug companies. As a result, (he claims) they ignored early warning signs of problems with Vioxx (Merck denied the allegation). If Senator Grassley had identified specific information of illegal behavior, he should have made it public

and prosecuted. If we needed corrective legislation, he should have introduced it.
2. The media loved Dr. Graham's congressional testimony alleging FDA misconduct. Government bashing helps sell advertising. In his testimony about Vioxx, he expressed concern for five other drugs. Acutane for acne has carried drug warnings since its debut. Merida for weight loss has comparable warnings. The three other drugs mentioned by Dr. Graham do have appropriate labeling and monitoring. In my opinion, nothing Dr. Graham said was new or alarming. The media generated all kinds of hype and nothing positive emerged for the future.
3. I graduated medical school in 1957 and was fully conversant with the Physician's Desk Reference (PDR). It was easy to look up drug information; indications for use, dosage, side effects and special considerations and precautions. I was taught way back then…know all there is to know about a drug before you prescribe it. With today's fingertip technology, it is easier than ever to do just that; as well as giving the patient a print-out, after discussing all

the ramifications of the condition you are treating.
4. The Kansas City Star carried an article in late December, 2004 about Republican Lousiana congressman, Billy Tauzin. He ran a congressional committee with responsibility to oversee the pharmaceutical industry. TV's 60 Minutes also interviewed him when, in 2005, he left congress to become CEO of Pharmaceutical Research and Manufacturers of America (PhRMA). Public interest groups, like Nader's Common Cause, contend Tauzin used his legislative position to line his own pockets. Listening to his interview on 60 Minutes, I would agree with Common Cause. He was not brought up on charges, and nothing was done to discourage such behavior in the future.
5. In 1992, congress passed the Prescription Drug User Fee Act which required pharmaceutical companies to pay for FDA processing of drug applications. Dr. Sidney Wolfe alleges conflict of interest; i.e. drug companies providing money for FDA oversight. He wants taxpayer money appropriated for FDA review of drug applications and follow-up. He claims this

would give the FDA true independence. I think we can appoint an independent oversight committee without eliminating funding from pharmaceutical companies.

6. Merck pulled Vioxx off the shelf September 30, 2004 following a review of crucial data. Merck alleges it paid for the monitoring of Vioxx, didn't conceal or delay release of adverse clinical findings, and asked to keep Vioxx in the market with a black box warning. The president of Merck testified before congress that his own wife had been on Vioxx right up to September 29, 2004. Pfizer's Celebrex (also a COX-2 medication) has remained with a black box warning, but Pfizer's other COX-2, Bextra, was removed from the market. Allegations and lawsuits proliferated and linger.

7. January 17, 2008: Allegations against Merck and Schering-Plough hit the media alleging that Vytorin (a combination of two drugs (Zetia and Mevacor) were no better than statins alone. My personal clinical experience is that Vytorin does do a better job in lowering cholesterol than *some* statins. Does it lower heart attack or stroke rates; did the drug companies make that claim? I'm not sure about either

question. The media embraced a chance for institution bashing and class action lawyers filed the following day. This does not provide an environment for meaningful investigation, or productive progress.

American's life expectancy increased to a record 77.3 years in 2002. Deaths from heart disease, cancer and stroke (the three leading adult killers) were all down 1-3 percent. The pharmaceutical industry has had a lot to do with increasing our longevity and quality of life. Some claim they're making too much money and would like to regulate them like a public utility. We could write another book about the pros and cons of governmental regulation of private enterprise. I suggest we give serious thought before over-regulating an industry that has given us so much.

Here's an example of doing appropriate investigation of legitimate questions. Diuretics have been used by millions of people to lower high blood pressure and reduce the long-term risks of death from heart attacks, strokes and kidney disease. Some diuretics, which work by removing fluid and salt from the body, carry a risk of promoting the onset of diabetes. Diabetes is, itself, a risk factor for cardiovascular disease. Did the risks of using certain diuretics cancel out the benefits? The first long-term study to examine this question was published in the January 2005 issue of the American Journal of Cardiology. The study was partly funded by the National Institute on Aging and the Robert Wood Johnson Foundation, and sponsored by the National Heart, Lung and Blood Institute.

It found that, while certain diuretics did raise the risk of developing diabetes, the rate of heart attacks and strokes was nearly 15 percent lower in patients getting a diuretic compared to those given placebos (dummy pills). Diuretics, one of medicine's oldest blood pressure drugs, cost just pennies a day. Some of the newer, more complex drugs, can cost up to 50 times more, have greater side effects and adverse drug interactions. <u>Lesson:</u> don't rush to new products when older products can do the job.

It's the doctor's responsibility to accurately evaluate a patient's risk factors and thoroughly explain the risk/benefit options of a treatment plan. This should obviously include non-pharmacological options like diet, exercise, cessation of smoking and minimizing alcohol consumption. Many doctors draw up a written treatment contract for the patient's signature…I encourage this approach; understanding and partnership are essential to successful outcomes.

Direct–to-consumer advertising increases pharmaceutical sales. However, insufficient regulatory laws and/or weak enforcement have allowed questionable marketing practices. I often wonder why one company shows a male and a female sitting in separate bathtubs in the middle of nowhere (tubs not connected to plumbing) as it extols the virtues of its erectile dysfunction medication. It doesn't look very romantic, or practical, to me.

The pharmaceutical companies promised legislators they would scale back and/or curtail the practice...in lieu of having laws passed to prohibit the practice. Have you seen any changes? Pharmaceutical promotion in 2005 reached $29.9 billion in the United States. I'll address food additives, supplements and over the counter con games later in this chapter.

An article in the Las Vegas Sun newspaper, January 5, 2005, stated:

"FOR SOME, BANNED DRUGS ARE WORTH THE RISK"

It went on to describe a lady who wanted her Vioxx back. She had been taking the drug for five years and dreaded a return to aches and stiffness that Vioxx controlled. Her words:

"Vioxx was the best pain drug I had been on in 27 years."

She has a chronic condition called fibromyalgia. She now takes Celebrex. Pfizer left it on the market despite media pressure and lawyer threats. The patient and her doctor must fully know and understand what's written on the label and package inserts…it's called informed consent.

Dr. Robert Bucholz, president of the American Academy of Orthopedic Surgeons and chairman of the orthopedic surgery department at the University of Texas Southwestern Medical School in Dallas stated:

"I personally took Vioxx ever since it was released. It's the one anti-inflammatory I can take that doesn't upset my stomach. When that was taken off the market, I was personally disappointed. I've gotten my own personal supply of Vioxx, and I'm not about ready to destroy it. All life is a series of risks, and you've got to measure the risks versus the benefits. And that's true of any drug."

Another confused patient was quoted in the same article. He's 51 and has suffered for two decades from a condition that combined the flaky skin of psoriasis with joint inflammation and pain of arthritis. Without anti-inflammatory pain medication, he finds it very difficult to work as a mechanic and service station owner.

"If someone grabs my hand, it can put me down on my knees."

After trying all kinds of medications, he settled on Celebrex. When he heard in mid-December that Celebrex, like Vioxx, might be associated with increased risk of heart problems, he became concerned about what to do. In reality, he has to look at the dosage, his beneficial results, risk factors such as stomach ulcers, personal and/or family heart problems, smoking, diabetes, blood pressure and alternative options. A worthy physician will go over all the details so both can set a course of reasonable treatment.

For another eye-opener, I refer to an article in USA Today, January 14, 2005: "about 80 million aspirin tablets are consumed daily in the USA. Of those, 72 percent are taken for disease prevention and 28 percent are taken for pain." The article contained an aspirin timeline:

- 400 B.C.: In Greece, Hippocrates gave women willow leaf tea to relieve the pain of childbirth.
- 1823: In Italy, aspirin's active ingredient is extracted from willow and named salicin.
- 1897: In Germany, Bayer's Felix Hoffman develops and patents a process for

synthesizing aspirin. First clinical trials begin.
1899: Aspirin launched.
1930's: Bayer's patent runs out; aspirin goes generic.
2004: More than 100 million tablets consumed worldwide each year.

Aspirin has been *grandfathered* in; it never went through the stringent tests for today's drugs. Pharmacist Harold DeMonaco, senior editor for Harvard Health Publications stated:

"My guess is that if aspirin was launched in 2004, it would not be an over-the-counter drug. People have the misunderstanding that if you simply buy it without a prescription, it is completely safe to use. But every drug has side effects."

Occasional use of aspirin for headache or minor pain does not run appreciable risk for causing gastrointestinal irritation and/or bleeding. However, chronic use requires careful historical review with monitoring for adverse side effects. One other comment…aspirin is aspirin. Don't be fooled by brand name advertising. This is one case where cheaper is just as good. Enteric coated formulas, however, may not be effective. They're touted to cause less chance of intestinal irritation by delaying absorption until they're in the intestine. Some, however, never dissolve.

If the pharmaceutical industry's prescription drugs are as bad as the trial lawyers and hypesters would like you to believe, why aren't they howling at the essentially unregulated multi-billion dollar health food/supplement industry which is rampant with misleading and/or blatantly fraudulent marketing practices?

This industry covers an entire spectrum of junk science to no science; no effects to harmful effects, including adverse drug interactions. Look at the following run-down from an insert in a Las Vegas newspaper (January 2005). The end of the second page, <u>in fine print,</u> carried the notice: *PAID ADVERTTISING*. Their "ULTRA HERBAL COMPLEX" was being touted for Cholesterol Health, Prostate Health, Night-sweats, Hot flashes, Menopause, Sexual/Stamina performance (contains Horny Goat Weed). The ad advised the reader to ask their *health store professional* about other products for PMS Support and Balance, Blood Pressure, Hair-Skin-Nails and Mental Concentration.

Talk about innuendoes…the ad was made to look academically authoritative with clever, attention-getting, hot-button words. They throw out the hook and hope you'll bite; no studies or warnings.

How does one become a *health store professional*? Easy; get a small business loan, open a store, learn the jargon and perfect the art of selling snake oil, combining mass psychology principles with Madison Avenue promotional know-how. You're guaranteed a 30 percent satisfied customer base using placebo response statistics: i.e. you give anything to 100 people and tell them it will help whatever ails them. At least 30 percent (plus or minus) will report improvement. If you decide to go into this type of business, it helps if you ignore conscience or ethics.

The huckster ads cleverly mix scientific jargon with loads of garbage. <u>I DO NOT BELIEVE IN ANY OF THE FOLLOWING,</u> but look at their outrageous claims. I challenge anyone to produce credible scientific study, short term or long term, for any of these claims. My comments are in parentheses.

- **Astragalus** – Acts as a tonic to protect the immune system. Aids adrenal gland function and digestion. Increases metabolism, promotes healing, and provides energy to combat fatigue. (assuming it can do all these things, what about side effects or adverse drug interactions?)

- **Bee Pollen** – Effective for combating fatigue, depression, cancer and colon disorders. Bee pollen is an excellent source of energy. (so is sugar)
- **Bladderwrack** – Increases thyroid activity and absorbs water in the intestines to produce bulk. Used in the treatment of obesity. (what isn't used in the treatment of obesity? Sponges absorb water too.)
- **Capsicum** – Stimulates the production of gastric juices (if true, this could be bad in people with stomach ulcers and acid reflux), improves metabolism (how?), high in vitamin C (vitamin C is the cheapest vitamin around. Why not buy it directly?).
- **Citrus Aurantium** – Provides an energy boost (so does high doses of caffeine…. would you put high octane gas in your lawn mower?), suppresses appetite and increases metabolic rate and caloric expenditure (the marketers of grapefruit and grapefruit pills make the same unproven claims).
- **Echinacea** – Stimulates the immune system and increases the body's ability to resist infection (show me the study). A natural antibiotic (Define what you mean by

natural. A friend of mine, a retired one star Air Force General, swore by Echinacea until he almost died of pneumonia. Good thing he consulted a doctor when his big "E" didn't seem to be working).

- **Deodorized Garlic** – (The odor is 95 percent of why it is used). Has a rejuvenating effect on all body functions. Used for infection, elevated cholesterol levels, high blood pressure, diabetes. (Larry King, for a time, was hawking *GARLIQUE* brand—shame on him).
- **Ginkgo Biloba** – Increases blood flow to the brain (so does pornographic movies) resulting in an increase in oxygen and glucose utilization (if this is true, it could be dangerous with a bleeding type of stroke).
- **Ginger Root** – A good digestive aid, helps relieve upset stomachs (so does reducing intake of spicy foods, alcohol and cessation of smoking).
- **Gotu Kola** – Aids in elimination of excess fluids, shrinks tissues, decreases fatigue, depression and increases sex drive. Used for mental disorders, high blood pressure, rheumatism, urinary tract infections, insomnia and stress (how about predicting the weather?).

- **Guarana** – Increases mental alertness and fights fatigue (should be good for all-night gamblers and party-goers).
- **Hyssop** – Used as a valuable cleansing agent for the lungs and throat (how does it do it, and where does the waste go? Sounds like a douche for the respiratory system?)
- **Licorice Root** – Pain reliever, exhibits hormone-like effect (what hormone?) Has been used to cleanse the colon (Exlax is more reliable).
- **Magnolia Extract** – Alleviates stress, reduces anxiety and depression (must be a Southern thing).
- **Myrrh** – Valuable as a cleansing and healing agent to the stomach and colon (Americans have a morbid fixation with the stomach and bowels).
- **Phosphatidylserine** (pronouncing it is a test in itself) Reduces cortisol levels and helps keep memory related pathways functioning smoothly (some things are best forgotten).
- **Rehmannia Root** – The herb is used to treat anemia (what kinds of anemia?), fatigue and to promote the healing of injured bones.

- **Reishi Mushroom** – Helps stimulate liver activity and lower stress (in the real medical world, anything that could 'stimulate' the liver requires close laboratory monitoring, like the Statin drugs that lower blood cholesterol).
- **Rhodiola Rosea** – helps stimulate the nervous system (the street calls such things *UPPERS OR SPEED*, amphetamines have been longtime favorites). Enhances work performance (the government should provide it for legislators and beaurocrats.
- **Siberian Ginseng** – Increases sexual functions, stamina, and is good energy source (they tell me Siberian tigers are quite horny).
- **White willow Bark** – Fever reducer and alleviates pain (what's wrong with generic aspirin? It's the same ingredient, and much purer).

As you can see, this partial list suggests endless panaceas, and mentions no risks or precautions. The same flier gave the following indictment of pharmaceutical companies while touting the superior benefits of natural herbs. My comments continue in parentheses.

"Many plants contain compounds that have a high degree of medicinal value (always give credibility to your statements by opening with a general touch of truism). It is generally known that for the past 25 years, 25 percent of all prescription drugs sold in the United States have contained active ingredients obtained from plants (I'd like to know what study showed this? Even if true, which I seriously doubt, so what?). In 1980 alone, Americans paid more than $8 billion for prescription drugs obtained from plants (Again, what is the source of this revelation... and so what? What about the FDA process for licensing drugs; i.e. safety, efficacy and benefit beyond current treatments. The industry doesn't just squeeze a plant and sell the juice. There are hucksters that do just that, but not with FDA approval).

Since a plant cannot be patented (this is totally false) very little research has been done this century on plants for medicinal value by the large American pharmaceutical firms (a blatant lie). Since a crude herb provides no economic reward to these firms, the crude herb never reaches the market place (three lies in a row should invoke a life sentence behind bars. The real world of legitimate medicine does not sanction Harry Potter-like potions and concoctions)."

The incredible gullibility of Americans with its resultant consequences were shown in a November 22, 2004 Las Vegas Review Journal article entitled:

COMPANY TOUTS PILLS FOR MIDDLE AGE MIDDLE CLASS

The subtitle read, "Dietary supplement peddler faces class action lawsuit, thousands of complaints over vague promises." This is a citizen/consumer initiated legal action. Why don't we have laws and enforcement from State and Federal arenas?

The recipient of the class action suit is Steven Warshak, president of Berkeley Premium Nutraceuticals (clever title for a company), who reportedly was taking in over $200 million per year on unproven palliatives for virtually every malady of the 'middle-age middle class'.
Mr. Warshak started out by selling Enzyte, *his natural male enhancement,* an alleged penis enlarger and virility booster pill (imagine that.... two fantasies for the price of one). He did so well with this gimmick, he went on to market Avlimil… the female equivalent sex enhancer; Dromias for insomnia, Altovis for fatigue, Numovil to fight memory loss, Rogisen for deteriorating vision and Rovicid to lower cholesterol.

Despite being the defendant in a class action lawsuit and the target of more than 3000 complaints to the Better Business Bureau, he continued to market his products and laugh all the way to the bank.

Unlike drugs that must be proven safe and effective before they can be sold, nutritional supplements and food additives are largely exempt from the FDA process. They can't claim cures but they can use clever advertising to suggest unsubstantiated possibilities. Penalties are rare and if enacted, are worth the huge profits.

In October 2004, the FDA sent Warshak a letter demanding he stop claiming Rovicid can lower cholesterol and prevent heart disease. The letter also objected to marketing Prulato for the prevention of prostatic cancer and Rogisen for preventing macular degeneration. The FDA should have taken him to court, and legislators should have closed the loopholes and enacted very severe penalties for such predators.

Caveat emptor, buyer beware: read the fine print and don't let fantasy create denial. Risk versus benefit applies to every aspect of daily living. You have a responsibility to be realistic, informed, reasonably critical and healthfully skeptical.

After fifty years of experience in healthcare, I continue to recommend NOT using a newly released medication unless it represents something uniquely innovative and vitally necessary to your well being or survival. Wait a few years and see how it does in 'the real world'. Clinical research, as it is currently practiced, raises many concerns about the validity of reported results. Don't volunteer or share medications with your friends or relatives, or try off-label experimentation. Here is an example that emphasizes the point.

Our youngest son is an anesthesiologist with a hospital-based group, affiliated with a Midwestern medical school. They signed on to clinically evaluate Bextra (Pfizer's COX-2 anti-inflammatory, pain-killer) for patients undergoing coronary bypass operations for blocked arteries supplying the heart muscles. It was doing a great job controlling postoperative pain, and the anesthesia department had lots of it sitting around. My son had symptoms of plantar fascitis; pain along the sole of one foot. He put himself on Bextra and it did make his foot feel better…so would lots of other anti-inflammatories. A few weeks later he experienced classic chest pain, which turned out to be caused by a blockage of a small artery on the backside of the heart. This happened while at work in the hospital. Quick recognition and prompt treatment resulted in minimal heart damage.

Our son had no cardiac risk factors; negative family history on both sides, non-smoker, lean weight, no diabetes, normal cholesterol patterns, physically active and normal blood pressure. Bextra had to be the cause of his heart attack. I urged him to report the incident to Pfizer so that it would be put into their database. There was no intention to sue or blame Pfizer. He had taken it upon himself to use an unlicensed, experimental drug for 'off-label use'. Shortly after that incident, Bextra was withdrawn from investigational trials because of increased cardiac risk associated with its usage.

A reporter in Las Vegas, Marshall Allen, deserves a Pulitzer Prize for medical investigative reporting. Among other things, his 2008 newspaper articles illuminated detailed flaws in professional medical licensing, blatant malpractice, abuse of foreign doctors with J-1 visas and the explosive misuse of prescription drugs. His hard work once again confirmed the fact that we have many good physicians and institutions…BUT…. the SYSTEM is totally broken when it comes to affordable, reliable, accessible, responsible scrutiny. It's all readily evident and the failure to take corrective action points the accusing finger to all members of our collective society...patients, providers, legislators and judicial practitioners. If you choose not to get informed and speak up, then others will act in their interests, not yours.

CHAPTER V

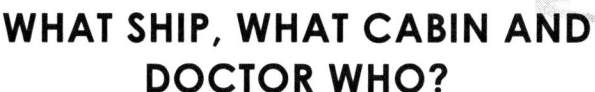

WHAT SHIP, WHAT CABIN AND DOCTOR WHO?

Not enough attention is given to medical services when people decide to travel, especially on cruise ships. I got first hand knowledge when I became a cruise ship physician (1990 to 1994). Having grown up on the East Coast, I enjoyed the pleasures of beaches and salt water. Living in Las Vegas for over 35 years has not diminished the call of the sea.

I had just left my 18-year position as Medical Director for the Nevada Atomic Test Site and was leafing through a family practice medical journal in the library of the teaching hospital. An ad for a ship's physician caught my attention. An emergency group out of Baltimore, Maryland had contracted for the medical services of the Regent Lines, under the contract name of Maritime Medical Services.

The Regent Lines had five ships of 1960's vintage (The Regent Sun, The Regent Sea, The Regent Rainbow, The Regent Spirit and The Regent Star). A Greek man had bought the ships, refitted them and contracted out many of the ship's services, like medical and food. The cabins were spacious, the food and entertainment was good, itineraries were interesting and prices were very competitive. The owner was apparently well trained in deficit financing; he kept the subcontractors and investors dangling while he siphoned off a good part of the cash flow. The operation went bankrupt in 1995.

I applied for the job…after getting an enthusiastic okay from my wife. Our children had left the nest and she relished the idea of joining me for romantic adventure in domestic and foreign ports. After waiting several weeks for a reply, I decided to call and see if I was still being considered for a job.

A gravelly-voiced female with a distinctive asthmatic wheeze answered the phone. After saying *Maritime Medical,* she went into a series of wet coughs, and paused to catch her breath.

"Oh yes," she said. "I remember your application. Glad you called. We happen to be looking for someone just like you. Can you be ready to travel by next week?" she asked.

I welcomed the assignment and we became good telephone buddies. I accepted the reality of dealing with a loosely run business model. I also encouraged my newly found Maritime

Medical friend to stop smoking. I subsequently became an aficionado of cruising…. as a ship's physician, as a passenger and as a guest lecturer.

Most cruise lines contract out medical services. For example, the Crystal ships use a medical group out of Sweden. I once met the head of that group while cruising as a passenger on the Crystal Symphony. I asked if he hired American physicians?

"Yes, we did hire an American once, but he lived in Sweden."

The Renaissance Lines, before going bankrupt, contracted with a Hispanic physician out of Florida. He hired doctors from Central and South America. Holland America (before its takeover by Carnival Cruises) ran its own medical service. At the time, in my opinion, it had the best screening process and consequently the best prospect for quality shipboard medical care in the cruise industry. Carnival took over Holland America, but it still sails under its brand name. We took the Ryndam, a Holland ship, roundtrip from San Diego to the Sea of Cortez, in early 2008. I chatted with the ship's doctor; a well-qualified internist from U.C. Davis. He assured me the Holland Line only hired American and Canadian physicians. The Ryndam, on that cruise, appeared to have very good medical coverage; not true for the industry as a whole.

My observation is that, in general, medical recruiters for cruise lines prefer foreign nationals. They work cheaper and are less problematic in the litigious arena. Who would you sue if a problem arose and the medical supplier was an independent contractor? An event could most likely occur in international waters or in a foreign port, with a foreign-trained, foreign national physician. If you read your cruise contract papers, you might be surprised to see a ship's disclaimer for medical care responsibility.

Next time you take a cruise, look at the nationalities of the ship's crew: musicians, deck hands, officers and hotel staff. There are usually between 35 and 50 different nationalities represented on a medium-sized cruise ship (1500 passengers). THERE ARE NO MANDATORY STANDARDS for physicians or nurses. Ships going in and out of United States ports have to comply with safety and health regulations, but there are no required educational or competency standards for medical personnel. Many lines would stay out of American ports if they could; thus avoiding U.S. Coast Guard inspections. Some smaller lines, like those in the Mediterranean, never do venture past the straight of Gibraltar.

I'd encourage you to check health and safety details before planning a *dream vacation* confined to distant parts of the world.

Most ships are registered in places other than the United States, for economic and political/legal reasons. So, you can roll the dice, pick a cruise and hope for the best….or….you can seek answers to pertinent questions…and then hope for the best.

Cruise insurance comes in all sizes and shapes. Travel magazines recommend third party coverage. If you insure with the cruise line, the coverage could be as worthless as the line, should they declare bankruptcy and leave you stranded. This happened with the Regent Line (where I had worked), and later with the Renaissance Line. Always read the fine print before buying medical coverage and/or cruise cancellation/delay. For example, will your insurance cover expensive air evacuation, should the need arise? Conde' Nast and Travel+Leisure magazines have good recommendations for insurance coverage.

When the captain has his welcome aboard party, the usual rhetorical question is: *"who's sailing the ship?"* The actual work of running the ship falls to the Staff Captain and his officers, deck hands and ship's crew. The Captain has the ultimate responsibility and he (I haven't seen a female cruise ship captain yet) usually has an impressive list of career credentials. Everything related to passenger services comes under the control of the Hotel Manager and his staff (housekeeping, food services, bar and beverage, entertainment, laundry, shore excursions, concierge, purser's office and medical. Some of these departments may be subcontracted, but the Hotel Manager still oversees the delivery of passenger services and reports to the Captain.

    Passengers would be amazed by the contrasting living conditions of the crew. The newer ships are much better than the older ships. I made a crew cabin call on one of my 60's vintage Regent ships where I walked past laundry hanging in the alleyway, bulkheads in desperate need of paint and gross over crowding. It looked like photos from a New York East Side tenement building in the early 1900's. A deckhand was recovering from Chickenpox. Four crewmen shared a 150 square foot cabin with two bi-level bunks.

    Another time, on an Alaskan run out of Vancouver, I wandered into the crew's galley. They were very surprised and pleased to have the doctor, in his white jacket and scrub suit, grace them with his presence. It apparently was the first time a ship's doctor had taken time to visit their work and living areas. A good share of their food was ethnic (central American and Asian): lots of rice and beans, deep-fried everything, dried fish, high calorie staples with liberal quantities of hot sauces and spices. I took a peak into a huge pot on a large stove. Salmon fish heads were bubbling in some sort of vegetable stew.

"Where's the rest of the salmon?" I asked the head chef.

"On the passenger tables, not here," smiled the Filipino galley veteran.

The crew doesn't starve, but they certainly don't eat from the top of the menu. They frequently worked 12 or more hours per day, in 6 to 12 month segments. They made good money by comparison to where they called home, and they earned every penny of it.

A Chinese crew ran the laundry on the Regent ships. The head man spoke passable English, but his crew spoke little to no English. They ate in the laundry area and I never saw them mingling with the rest of the crew. One laundry worker came for medical care for a persistent hand rash. I shocked the hell out of them when I descended into the forward bowel of the ship to inspect their working conditions and laundering products. Communication was difficult, but I managed to convey the message that I wanted the man with the hand rashes to wear protective gloves or be transferred to a detergent-free area in the laundry. Keeping him on long-term cortisone creams was not acceptable. The head man was very appreciative of my personal interest and unprecedented visit to the ship's laundry. I received free laundry service for the remainder of my cruise.

Ships have histories and personalities. The Regent Sun, for example, was built by the Germans and given to Israel as part of World War II reparations. It was renamed the SHALOM. The Israeli's never did get the hang of running a cruise ship; they lost money and had a few mishaps.

The ship ran on diesel fuel and reportedly used 180 gallons to travel one mile…how's that for global warming? They had very limited capability for desalination. Consequently, we bought fuel and water at just about every port of call. The engine rooms were about as close to Hollywood's version of hell as you can get: located deep down in the ship, constantly over 100 degrees Fahrenheit with deafening sound levels. The crew was issued sound mitigating ear coverings that hung, unused, around the work areas.

The Greek engineers sat inside an air-conditioned, remarkably quiet, windowed room from which they could view the important areas of the engine complex. The Indonesian and Filipino deck hands worked in the noisy, very hot, dirty, oily, hands-on areas of the engine room. I tapped one of the men on his shoulder and pointed to the hearing protectors hanging on a nearby pole. He smiled and shrugged. Most of these men were hearing impaired. I thought back to my training as a specialist in Occupational and Environmental Medicine, and OSHA's (Occupational Safety and Health Association) standards for noise, heat and air quality. Dream on: different lines undoubtedly had different degrees of conscience and compliance to worker's compensation guidelines, but the Regent Line was back in the dark ages. Here are several medical case examples from my experiences at sea.

I certainly didn't sign on for the money. Maritime Medical, the company that paid my salary, gave me $200 per week plus ten percent of charges for passenger medical care. I received no money for crew medical care. Regent Lines did pay Maritime Medical for crew visits. I don't know whether they got a lump sum for crew care, per visit pay, or both? I paid for my own airfare to and from the ship's port, unless they called me on short-notice emergency coverage. I paid for my wife's airfare if she came along, as well as her port charges. We got a cabin, meals, use of the facilities and were asked not to gamble or compete in passenger contests.

The casino concession was run by a British company. I understand Regent was guaranteed $10,000 plus a percentage of the take for each 7-10 day cruise: Regent couldn't lose.

I had office hours from 8:00 to 10:00 AM, after which I saw crew members. I also had scheduled office hours in the late afternoon from 4:00 to 6:00 PM. My nurse and I were available 24/7 and we took turns being on call nights and during port stops. We had approximately 900 passengers and an equal number of crew. Many passengers were upset to learn that medical care was not covered in the cost of the cruise. A visit, or cabin call, carried a base price and medications, tests (like EKG or urine analysis) and extra time carried additional charges. I considered the fee schedule very reasonable. Nevertheless, some passengers would forego medical care to save money. It never made sense to me; i.e. they're spending thousands of dollars for a vacation, why stint on medical care that might ruin their vacation...or even put their life in jeopardy. Go figure human priorities.

The demands for passenger medical services were usually minimal, unless we hit stormy weather. Taking care of the crew could be more demanding in time, communication, medical emergencies and social interactions. One had to be ready for all types of situations.

My wife and I boarded the Regent Sun in Ft. Lauderdale, Florida and settled in for a 10 day Caribbean cruise. The first port was San Juan, Puerto Rico. The seas became a little rough as we started our two day run to San Juan. I got a request for a cabin visit. A wife suspected her husband was reacting poorly to the rolling and pitching of the ship. The nurse asked the wife if she would consider bringing the husband down to the medical clinic to avoid the extra charge of visiting their cabin. No, she wanted us to come up, and as soon as possible.

The poor man was sitting in bed, whiter than his sheets. He appeared confused about time and place, and was having trouble focusing as I introduced my nurse and myself. It didn't take long to determine he was experiencing double vision, difficulty in coordinating his arm movements and was not able to carry on a logical conversation. I took the wife aside and asked about his medical history since this was not a characteristic picture of motion sickness.

Turns out he was diagnosed with lung cancer a few months prior to this cruise. His doctor had made him 'more comfortable' prior to their sailing by removing a few quarts of liquid from his chest...she matter-of -factly volunteered. GREAT! I would have liked having his doctor on board so that he could take care of this man who, in my opinion, should have never been allowed to go on this cruise.

I informed the wife what she should have known (maybe she <u>was</u> told and chose to ignore it?); her husband had lung cancer in various parts of his body (including metastases to brain) which caused his current problems; not motion sickness. I outlined a plan for trying to make her husband more comfortable during the next two days at sea. She would then have two options when we got to San Juan.

I told her we could move him to one of our two beds in the medical department, or we could start treatment in the cabin and see how he did with periodic visits. The nurse outlined the fees she could expect, and we got signed agreements for everything. She opted for the cabin trial.

We started intravenous fluids, patched one eye for visual comfort and gave him medication for nausea. I then took an educated guess: I figured his mental status was probably due in some degree to brain inflammation and swelling caused by the metastatic lung cancer. I added sizeable amounts of cortisone to his intravenous fluids with the hope of decreasing reactive brain inflammation. The nurse and I drew up a schedule for periodic cabin visits, and on-call availability for possible emergencies. I informed the Hotel Manager and the ship's Captain of the situation. It was fine with them, as long as it didn't require diverting or disrupting the ship's planned itinerary.

By the next morning, I was ready to light a candle (not normal for a minimally observant Jewish boy) and make a donation. The man was remarkably better. I humbly accepted the praises and thanks of the wife, while I crossed my fingers and toes, with the hope he would remain improved long enough to get on a plane in San Juan and head home. Her two options, once we got to San Juan, was to board a commercial flight and head home (if we could get seats), or check into a local hospital and make arrangements from there. God smiled. She was a travel agent and arranged for two first class seats. A private charter flight would have cost over $20,000. We assisted with the transfer to the airport, and arranged for medical care upon their New York arrival. I asked if she could drop me a note about their trip back. I never heard from her, but fellow passengers for the remainder of the cruise told me they got word they had made it back okay and appreciated the care given aboard ship.

    Maritime Medical did not like their doctors or nurses purchasing supplies on their own. They obviously saved money by bulk buying through discount houses, notably pharmaceuticals through generic Canadian suppliers. I called Maritime Medical from San Juan because we had used most of our supply of intravenous solutions and were out of a few other medications. They promised to have supplies waiting at our next port. I was skeptical about the promise. I had noticed signs of discord between the Hotel Manager and my bosses at Maritime Medical. In retrospect, it was subcontract problems that would eventually lead to declaration of bankruptcy by the Regent Line. I was planning to purchase a few supplies in San Juan and charge them to the Maritime account in the purser's office.

Our dock space was facing the old city of San Juan, not far from the El Morro fortress. Parked next to us was a United States cruiser resting from its patrol duties around Haiti. I donned my scrub suit, white jacket with name tag, and requested permission to board the cruiser and visit its doctor (this was way before 9/11). I was informed the ship only carried corpsmen; no doctor. They put in a call and asked me to wait at the head of the gangplank. I was soon greeted by a young corpsman…ready, able and proud to show me around his ship. As we exchanged medical stories, with added information about his ship's fighting capabilities, I mentioned my supply problems.

"No sweat, Doc, I can give you all the fluids you want, but we'll have to see how much reserve I have for the medications you need."

It turned out great. I got all the supplies I needed and in turn I invited all three corpsmen, and a few of their friends, for dinner aboard the Regent Sun. None had been on a civilian cruise ship before. They were duly impressed with the people comforts, and they surprised me with their menu selections. My assumption had been that our fighting men and women had an abundance of the best when it concerned food. I diplomatically asked about their selections of lobster and steak They told me their budgets had been cut back (sound familiar?) which spilled over to limited commissary supplies. Incidentally, no supplies were waiting at our next port, as promised by Maritime Medical.

One of my last trips as a ship's physician was again on the Regent Sun, out of New York City. My wife and I looked forward to an October cruise up the East Coast. We sailed past New York's majestic evening skyline, waved to Miss Liberty and proceeded on to Provincetown, Portland, Bar Harbor, Montreal, Quebec and Nova Scotia. As we made our return approach to New York in early November, I was asked if I could make the Sun's last roundtrip to the Caribbean before its repositioning for the winter months. We decided that my wife would get off the ship and return home, and I would make the 12 day southern roundtrip. The U.S. rule is that any ship with 100 or more passengers, had to have a physician aboard. I was doing the Sun a big favor.

I sensed we were in trouble the minute we cleared New York heading south. A storm had come up the coast and the ship started to pitch, roll and slam into rising waves. I suggested the Hotel Manager ask the Captain to modify the usual lifeboat drill. I thought it wise to inform passengers to skip the drill if they were medically and/or physically not up to it. We did have a predominantly elderly population. The Hotel Manager felt such an announcement was redundant. I later concluded he was reluctant to advise the Greek Captain, or the Captain's First Officer (the Captain's German wife) of anything. They would turn out to be the worst bridge officers of my short sailing career. Thank God for the Italian Staff Captain. He was pleasant and always ready to help the nurse or myself.

    We went into a terrible storm, and the lifeboat drill added to the casualties. We had people slipping, tripping and falling…plus 120 or so calls for nausea and vomiting, in the first two hours at sea. At one point the nurse counted 21 people in our little two-room medical complex. We were injecting phenergan and advising bed rest and fluids as fast as we could. At one point I was considering sending a contingent of *pewkers* up to vomit all over the Hotel Manager and his Captain. The nurse and I were one tired duo as we docked at our first port, Aruba. The calm, warm Caribbean Sea was welcomed by everyone.

    The nurse and I were enjoying a pre-dinner drink with friends in a forward lounge. We received an emergency call from the first seating in the main dining room. The ship had left Curacao and was on its way to St. Thomas, U.S. Virgin Islands; its last stop before heading back to New York for dry dock and winter repositioning.

As we entered the crowded dining room, we spotted the group we were looking for in a far corner of the room. A very large man was lying motionless on the floor while a passenger was attempting resuscitation. Observers were offering opinions and advice. One, very intoxicated female was standing nearby, shouting….

"Get up you son of a bitch, I'm not flying home by myself."

It so happened this was the man's second wife, married to the brother of a very well known American comedian. The nurse became quite annoyed by the crowd blocking access to the patient. I could see the patient was cyanotic (very blue lips and ashen-gray complexion) with no signs of life. I advised the nurse to call for a stretcher and a few strong attendants to help us remove the man to the infirmary. The stretcher arrived with four muscular Jamaicans. We quickly loaded and left.

The deceased was in his seventies but looked ninety. He was loaded with all kinds of jewelry; gold and diamond rings, gold necklaces with one huge door-knocker size golden pendant, gold bracelets and a Rolex watch. His cuff-linked shirt was unbuttoned to his mid-chest. He looked like a stereotyped Las Vegas high roller commonly seen during the Rat Pack years. He was 6 foot 4 inches and at least 75 pounds overweight. He smelled of vomit, cigarettes, cigars and liquor. There wasn't much doubt he died of an acute myocardial infarction (heart attack).

The intoxicated wife arrived shortly after we managed to get him and the stretcher onto the examining table. He was too heavy to lift off the stretcher. She circled the body a few times before asking if she could give him one last farewell kiss. Who could refuse such a tender request? She then proceeded to remove all his jewelry (we noted the event into his written record with date, time and itemized articles).

The staff captain told me the one-body cooler was on the top deck (10 flights above us). He had turned it on before coming down to medical. It would take at least two hours to completely cool down. You might ask what would we have done if we had gotten another body or two? No problem; the staff captain informed me we could have put them in the food lockers…in body bags of course.

The new widow left with the hotel manager. We wrapped two sheets around the body and stretcher, and secured them with canvas straps. He was just too big to try placing into a body bag. The nurse and I then left for the hotel manager's office. I tried to answer the widow's irrelevant questions as they placed a call to the deceased's son in Riverside, New York. The widow grabbed the phone as soon as contact was made.

"Your dad finally bought the farm. Doc says he didn't suffer. Now listen; I don't want (she rattled off a list of names) at the fucking funeral. Bullshit, I'm here alone. I have the final say. Here, Doc, he wants to talk to you." She handed me the phone.

The first question to me was:

"Is my stepmother drunk again?"

We had an intelligent discussion. He informed me that his dad had had two previous heart attacks. He was a diabetic, overweight, hypertensive, heavy smoker and drinker and determined to do it his way…right to the end. We gave him the protocol for having the body flown back from St. Thomas and he thanked us for our efforts. The nurse and I never got paid for our efforts, and we decided not to pursue it.

Almost four hours had passed since our patient's demise. It was after midnight. The nurse and I left the hotel manager's office and returned to the medical infirmary. We had to move the body to the cooler on the top deck. The nurse offered four Jamaican cabin attendants $5 each to act as stretcher-bearers. We decided the easiest most direct route would be to head for the nearest opening to the rear deck and up the outside set of stairs. Somehow the hotel manager got involved, and insisted on a set of inside, tortuous staircases. He reasoned that his route was least likely to encounter late night passengers. I wondered how many senior citizens would be wandering around the outside decks after midnight? He outranked us, so up the inside we went.

The Jamaicans struggled with the heavy load on the narrow, winding stairways. After negotiating two levels, they stopped to assess a strong fecal odor permeating the stairwell. The body, with all the food and liquor inside, had been lying around for four hours at room temperature. Fermentation was creating gas, bloating and odors. The Jamaicans looked at each other, wondering if one of them had passed gas. They all denied causing the problem.

"Not me, maaan!" was the emphatic refrain.

They scrutinized the body wrapped in sheets. As if on cue, the corpse 'burped' fluid which produced a gurgling sound and a wet stain on the sheet in the vicinity of the mouth. The four men dropped the stretcher and pulled back in horror.

"Da maaan is arguing wid da devil", exclaimed one of the Jamaicans.

Only two could be coaxed back…. by offering an additional $10 each. The nurse and I each took hold of a corner of the stretcher. We finally made it to the cooler and called it a night.

The funeral people were waiting at the dock in St. Thomas. We arrived around 8:00 AM. The staff captain was preparing to use the side arm designed for the specific purpose of swinging the stretcher and body clear of the top deck and lowering it directly down to the dock. The hotel manager once again intervened, saying that it might attract unwanted passenger attention. He directed the body again be taken down through inside staircases. At that point I grabbed the nurse's arm and left the scene. I later heard that someone had removed the straps securing the body and sheets to the stretcher. The body rolled off the stretcher at least once before making it to the dock.

It wasn't long before I wondered if someone had buried an albatross in the hold of the Regent Sun. Departure from St. Thomas was tentatively delayed 12 hours. They hoped they could fix one of the main boilers. It was essential for providing hot water for the laundry and passenger cabins. We finally left without a working boiler. I suspect Regent's credit line was beginning to crumble. A public announcement was made after we left St. Thomas; "expect limited hot food and very limited hot water for cabin use". I also heard that housekeeping had been short-changed by the contractor providing linen service in St. Thomas. He was most likely reacting to missed payments from the Regent's owner. The boiler problem also meant reduced speed for the return trip. With luck, we'd arrive 1-2 days later than scheduled.

Free drinks and a beautiful sunset temporarily kept everyone in a good mood. The nurse and I were watching St. Thomas disappear off our stern when the beeper went off. I went to a phone and called a number manned by Jamaican cabin attendants.

"Docteur, Docteur, day need ya at da aft elevator on deck 6."

I waved for the nurse to follow me, and proceeded to deck 6. The elevator in question was the size of a telephone booth. An elderly gentleman had gotten in (it could comfortably hold only one person) and had passed out. He couldn't fall to the floor because of the tight space, so his unconscious body lay erect against the elevator door. When the door opened, he fell forward and hit the floor with his face…still unconscious. His face showed signs of the impact with bruising and swelling, but he was breathing normally, had good color and a steady pulse. I asked the nurse to get our scoop stretcher. Guess what? The funeral people in St. Thomas had never returned our stretcher (I doubt it was an oversight). I remembered the old rusty stretcher we had pulled out of the cooler before putting in the deceased, wrapped into our relatively new clinic stretcher. We found the rusty relic, wrapped it in blankets to hide the shabby metal, and got our man to medical. His vital signs were remarkably stable. We located his wife; a 60-ish lady, definitely 20 years younger than her husband. She looked at the peacefully resting man with the bruised face and calmly said;

"He does this quite often. He gets some kind of irregular heart rhythm that causes him to pass out. He should come around shortly."

The man opened his eyes and looked around without moving his head, or other body parts. I asked if he was hurting anywhere?

He calmly replied, "No", but didn't move.

The nurse helped me sit him up. He smiled at his wife and prepared to get off the table. I gave him a careful examination and went over the signs and symptoms of head trauma he and his wife should monitor, before allowing him to leave. We documented everything and marveled at the resiliency of the human body.

Things were quiet for the next 48 hours and I thought that maybe the Albatross had left the ship. It was not to be; two more challenges were on the way.

I was watching the live, after dinner theater show when my beeper went off. I stopped by medical to pick up my doctor's bag and proceeded to cabin 1340. A very calm elderly gentleman opened the door and welcomed me in. His wife was sitting in bed, looking very tired but in no acute distress. The history was that aside from small amounts of water, she had not taken anything by mouth since leaving St. Thomas (we were going into our third day at sea). Nothing would stay down. Her temperature was normal. She was mentally clear. She had no pain except for slight discomfort with pressure to the center of her abdomen. She was not distended and her bowel sounds were normal. This was a puzzler. She had no significant past medical history.

I told her I'd like to check a urine sample and take some blood for a hemoglobin level. That was the extent of our laboratory capabilities. We had no x-ray machine or ultrasound equipment. I told the couple I could not give them a diagnosis, but we could start intravenous fluids and anti-emetics (nausea blocking medications). I advised ordering light foods and trying to eat at her convenience and tolerance. They were very cooperative and pleasant.

It was my night to be on call. I told the nurse I would periodically look in on our patient. I wouldn't call her unless I got very busy. The night went well. The patient was able to get 6 hours of sleep and felt better, but still not normal. She told me her son and daughter-in-law were both radiologists at a New York Hospital. I told them we would call when we were within a few hours of docking in New York. Her urine analysis did confirm ketosis and dehydration (lack of fluids and nourishment). Her hemoglobin level was normal. I encouraged movement about the cabin, and food as tolerated.

I notified the Hotel Manager of the situation in cabin 1340, and he handed me another problem. He asked me to come down to his office for a meeting with the ship's Security Officer.

An unmarried couple, traveling together, had been drinking quite heavily. The man was 10 to 15 years older than his traveling companion. The alcohol unleashed his mean streak. Neighbors complained of noise and suspected violence. The Security Officer took the battered, inebriated woman to a vacant lounge area. The couple had been noisy and disruptive from the beginning of the cruise, and it was getting progressively worse. The Security Officer was now concerned about serious harm to the woman. I suggested they keep the man in his cabin and bring the woman down to medical. I offered to sedate the man if he balked at confinement to his cabin.

The lady was in her late 50's and very drunk. Her clothes looked like she'd been sleeping in them for several days. Her nylon stockings were full of tears, hair disheveled and she smelled like leftover saloon yuck. I came up with the following plan.

I offered to have the nurse clean her up and get her into an infirmary bed. I'd start an intravenous (she certainly needed fluids) and I'd periodically add enough valium to keep her sleepy for the rest of the voyage. I planned to let her wake up 4-5 hours before docking in New York. I suggested telling her male companion, if he asked, that she was resting in a private cabin…doctor's orders. Both ship's officers were concerned about their liability. I promised to cover everything in the medical record; i.e. document that we'd taken the necessary action to protect these two patients from harming each other, as well as ensuring the health and safety of other passengers. We now had two patients on intravenous solutions; one in cabin 1340 and one in the infirmary. The nurse and I took turns covering the night hours.

We docked in New York at midnight; 12 hours late. No one was allowed to leave the ship until clearance early the next morning. New York City police stood guard on the pier.

We had called ahead for the woman in cabin 1340. Her children had an ambulance waiting when we docked. It was weird getting her off at that hour. The dock was deserted and dead quiet, except for the police and ambulance. The air was damp and the dock floor was wet and grimy. It was two levels below the terminal disembarkation ramp. It was like a subway tunnel scene for a Hitchcock movie. I gave the husband copies of all my medical notes and asked if he would give me a call once they made a diagnosis. I never heard from them. I thought she might have had some type of abdominal cancer.

    I stopped the intravenous and valium on my sleeping beauty patient and sent her back to her beau around 2:00 AM. She looked ten years younger and radiant as she left the ship around 10:00 AM that morning; hand in hand with her sobered sugar daddy. They could have passed as poster people for a senior honeymoon cruise….lovers without a care in the world. He paid the $1200 medical bill in cash. The nurse and I each got 10 percent of $1200.

    I called my wife to let her know I'd be late getting back to Las Vegas. I thanked the nurse for her help and she thanked me for helping her make the most money she'd ever made on any 10-day cruise. We earned it.

    Another interesting case developed on the first Spring, Alaskan cruise, aboard the Regent Star. We were 3 hours out of Vancouver heading north along the inward passage when I got an urgent call for one of the VIP cabins. I got my bag from medical and put in a call to have the nurse meet me at the cabin. A familiar, unwelcome odor greeted me as a frantic woman, with a Russian accent, opened the cabin door. The odor couldn't be anything but melena (stool mixed with relatively stagnant blood).

I remembered my first encounter with that type of mess; as a medical student making rounds on a cancer ward. Some things never leave you. I also remember leaving the ward in that first encounter to privately throw up in the men's room. This time I wasn't nauseous, and I wasn't happy either.

I followed the woman to the cabin's bathroom. I pushed open the door and confirmed my nose's diagnosis. An extremely pale male sat on a bathroom floor covered with an inch thick layer of black, tarry, extremely smelly gook. His face was soaked with perspiration as he leaned his head against the vanity. I gathered all the towels I could reach and laid a path to the patient. The nurse arrived, in shock. I told her to get a stretcher, additional muscle power and to notify housekeeping. I would later ask the Staff Captain for permission to open the cabin's portholes for ventilation.

The man had come to the United States from St. Petersburg, Russia, 8-years previously. He was a scientist, living in the San Francisco Bay area. He had no personally significant past history. However, one son had a history of bowel cancer at an early age. I offered as much encouragement as possible while we extracted and transported the man down to medical. His blood pressure was low; he was sweaty and he looked like bleached white laundry. We started two intravenous lines. His color improved within 45 minutes. I examined him from top to bottom, including a digital/rectal exam. The wife was still in shock and prayer, as her husband tried to sit up.

"Whoa, we're not done here," I said, as I eased him back on the examining table. "I am sure you were bleeding from something in your stomach or intestine. You will need tests to figure out exactly what caused the bleeding. I've replaced your circulating volume with fluids which has helped bring your blood pressure back up. I assume you have stopped bleeding for now, since your blood pressure, pulse and color have improved and appear stable. Our first stop is Juneau, another 24 hours of sailing. You could start to bleed again, and it could be very serious…even fatal. My first choice is to have the captain return to Vancouver and send you to the hospital."

The heavy accented Russian frowned. "What's your next choice?"

"You could sign a release stating you understand the risks, and choose to go on to Juneau. I will get laboratory tests in Juneau to assess your blood loss. If you've lost 25% or more of your normal blood volume, I will insist you leave the ship and fly back To San Francisco. If you have good residual blood readings and your vital signs remain stable, I will not insist on your leaving the ship….but you will have to sign another release."

A broad smile came over his face. His wife's face was not so happy. They had a heated exchange in Russian. He won. He made it clear (to me) that they'd planned this trip for many months; it was fully paid and he was going on come hell or high water. We drew up the papers, watched him for another hour and let him go back to his cabin in a wheelchair. I did put him on anti-acids, Cimetidine (Tagamet, an H2 stomach acid blocker) and light sedation at night; on the hunch that maybe his bleed was due to stomach ulcers? I limited his physical activity and ordered a bland diet. I again marveled at the resiliency of the human body, and this man's stubborn resolve. By that afternoon he was sitting on a chaise lounge on the pool deck…at least in the shade. He smiled and told <u>me</u> not to worry.

His wife shrugged. "You can't tell him anything."

His blood work in Juneau was border-line low. He signed releases and completed the cruise to Seward. I gave him copies of his medical record, advised immediate follow-up and requested he send me a note from San Francisco.

"Thank you, doctor, but I still have the two-week land portion of my vacation: Denali Park, a glacier and everything else. Don't worry, I'm doing fine."

I never got a letter from him. Every time someone says "don't worry" I think of him.

People frequently ask if my cruising experience had elements of the Love Boat TV series? TV does take liberties and is prone to exaggeration. However, people are after all, people. I had all kinds of problems among the ship's crew; romantic entanglements requiring medical help, on the job injuries and stress related problems. On one cruise in the Caribbean, a young lady (assistant purser) came to me with a fever of 104 and pain under her right ribcage. She overcame her embarrassment and told me she had had a termination of pregnancy in Curacao two weeks previously. I assumed they had perforated her uterus and she now had an abscess between her liver and diaphragm (separating the chest from the abdomen). I was able to bring the fever down with huge doses of intravenous antibiotics, and immediately flew her back to San Juan (her home) at the next port. My diagnosis was correct and she did well with appropriate surgery and follow-up.

    The most colorful Love Boat character was an unmarried Greek captain who rivaled Bill Clinton's womanizing persona. He literally had women in every port…as well as inland cities. I'll never forget the time he appeared on the bridge with nothing but a towel around his waist. We were maneuvering away from the dock in Tampa, Florida. A heavy wind threatened a collision with the pilings. I never knew why the Captain wasn't on the bridge with the Staff Captain when we prepared to get underway…as had always been the case. Maybe the Captain decided to shower off his most recent romantic encounter. In any event he appeared in his towel-sarong to shout orders and keep the ship from bumping the dock. The towel came off with the heated activity. He paid no attention to the exposure. A picture of that event would have made a great ad for a "bare-ass cruise with a bare-ass captain in the Caribbean."

This same Captain asked me to call one of his girl friends in Las Vegas. He asked me to give her his regards and:

"Ask her why she never writes or calls me? Ask her if she is mad at me?"

I did call and pass on the message that he would like to hear from her. Her response:

"You ask that S.O.B. why he never answered <u>my</u> letters."

She continued with a very explicit string of adjectives. Her shouting voice did not drown out the noise of children carrying on in the background. She took a deep breath and asked:

"Are you married?"

I replied in the affirmative and hung up; so much for being a nice guy.

Most cruises are very enjoyable, as evidenced by their popularity. It's up to you to pick itineraries that minimize exposure to weather problems; the right place at the right time of the year. Avoid ships with histories of substandard passenger services; use Google and travel magazines. **Be prepared with your own medicines and basic first aid supplies and knowledge if you plan to visit out of the way places. If you're going to roll the dice on a cruise, stack the odds in your favor.**

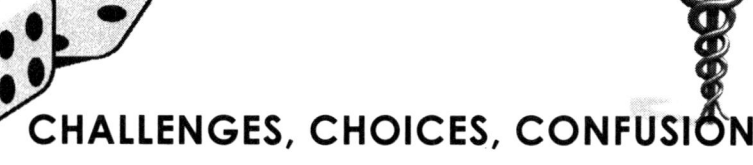

CHAPTER VI

CHALLENGES, CHOICES, CONFUSION

We'd all like to be free spirits; no rules, regulations or consequences. You and I know that's not the way it works. Approximately 40 percent of the United States health care dollars are directly traceable to the lifestyle consequences of alcohol and smoking. Throw in food abuse, misuse of prescription drugs, illegal drugs and sedentary lifestyles and the number easily goes over 50 percent. In other words, choosing to live like a jerk in perpetual denial and self-gratification accounts for major portions of health care costs in the United States, as well as a flawed healthcare system. Our leaders don't seriously address these issues because you, the consumers, aren't collectively concerned about it. When it affects you personally, you respond, sometimes. However, nothing will change until we ALL get riled up and off our collective asses.

The slogan, "What Happens in Las Vegas Stays in Las Vegas" should realistically say, "What Happens in Las Vegas Mirrors What's Happening

All Over The Country"…promoting and cashing in on fantasies and overindulgence.

Consider an actual example of Sin City advertsing: an oversized Las Vegas billboard showing a man lying on his back with his abdomen mounding up like Mount McKinley. The caption read:

"TODAY THE BUFFET, TOMORROW THE DIET" With coupons and practice, Las Vegans can find breakfasts in the $3 range, lunch for $5 and dinner for $7…. buffets to literally die for: gastronomy guaranteed to bring your weight and cholesterol to death-inviting levels.

If you gamble, and most people coming to Las Vegas do gamble, you get complimentary drinks, smokes and food. Complimentary is a relative term that comes with evidence of spending meaningful gaming time with the house. Computers track the action. There are literally no free lunches.

Las Vegas has exported its science of denial to proliferating casinos throughout the United States. Don't kid yourselves, the boys and girls of the Silver State have extensive financial tentacles and influence woven into the fabric of our country. I recommend you read, THE MONEY AND THE POWER by Denton and Morris.

I've seen very seedy, pathetic souls in Las Vegas casinos, especially in some of the older downtown establishments, who do not look like the TV commercials promoting the Mecca for fun and games.

Picture a person with chronic lung disease, cigarette dangling from pursed lips, clutching the sides of a slot machine, an oxygen canister at their side and prongs in their nostrils, gasping for air. The casinos know what people want and they supply it methodically and scientifically.

Our oldest son, as a college student in Reno, worked as a part time watchman for a company making gaming machines. He told us the company hired scientists to study the enticing effects of sound, visuals and odors: the bells, whistles and flashing lights are not random slot machine decorations. As little as possible is left to chance in the gaming world.

Smoking, drinking and eating are symbiotic to gambling. You do it to celebrate your winnings, and you do it to sooth depressive losings. Exploiting human weakness is not unique to Nevada and the gaming industry. USA Today carried an article at the end of December 2004 entitled: SM OKING MAKES THE CAMPUS SCENE. It went on to describe tobacco industry sponsored parties, complete with complimentary cigarettes. Here are statistics from the article.

1. Nearly one in ten college students have gone to an industry-sponsored party.
2. Students at all but one of the 119 colleges surveyed have attended the parties.
3. At some schools, 27% of students have attended tobacco bashes, that often include live music, and freebies such as T-shirts.
4. Students who did not smoke before college were almost twice as likely to start if they attended industry-backed parties that included free cigarettes.
5. Tobacco-sponsored events aim to link smoking with alcohol, music and socializing. Binge drinkers and marijuana users were more likely to attend these parties.
6. The rate of cigarette smoking declined from 1993-2000 among all adults, except ages 18-24.
7. Tobacco companies agreed not to market to anyone under 18 as part of the 1998 Master Settlement Agreement with 46 state attorneys general.
8. The tobacco industry is still clearly marketing to young adults as replacement smokers for ones dying off.

9. Spokesmen for R. J. Reynolds Tobacco and Phillip Morris USA dispute the allegation of supporting tobacco parties. Reynolds stated that it does give out cigarettes at bars and nightclubs that might be located near college campuses. Phillip Morris stated that it does not give out freebies, and both maintain they are only involved where proof of age 21 is provided. (Yeah, the same people who swore tobacco didn't cause cancer).
10. The American College Health Association suggests that colleges should not permit companies to give away tobacco products, such as cigarettes or smokeless tobacco, or to sponsor events on campus.

How many parents and grandparents seriously question these practices when sending their kids off to learn?

Despite what our Constitution says, all people are NOT created equal. None of us chose our parents. Our genetic bases differ, our metabolisms differ and the effects of environmental impacts differ. <u>WE DO, HOWEVER, HAVE LIFESTYLE CHOICES: DON"T SMOKE—IT'S PUBLIC ENEMY NUMBER ONE.</u> Drink in moderation, or not at all…especially if you have a family history of substance abuse and/or you are honest with yourself when it comes to evaluating dependency (your willpower). You can be the best judge when it comes to determining if you are *an easy mark*.

Put sensible exercise into your daily routine and set realistic goals when it comes to food. IT'S CALORIS IN VERSUS CALORIES OUT, no matter how the hucksters label it. Your body is the bank and foods are the deposits. Metabolic expenditures are the withdrawals. It's plain and simple math dealing with averages.

A United States female uses approximately 1500 to 1800 calories a day for routine activities of daily living (basic calorie expenditure). U. S. males burn 2000 to 2500 calories per day for basic caloric activity. These are averages; i.e. genetics accounts for some people using less calories for daily living, and some people using more calories. If you increase your activity (daily calorie use), and decrease your calorie intake, your body will have to burn stored calories (carbohydrates and fat) and you lose weight. Do the reverse and you gain weight.

Since all people are not created equal, some may have to work harder at losing than others. You can easily customize you body *bank account* by making a list of the calories you eat each day and determining what levels keep your weight steady, what levels allow weight loss and what levels add weight. You quickly learn which foods are best to avoid. All the branded diets like South Beach, Scarsdale, Slimfast, etc. are merely selling you prepackaged calorie amounts. You'll lose weight on most of them, if you stick to the allowed amounts. It may be easier than selecting your own foods, determining the caloric content and doing your own math…but it is definitely more expensive, and some preparations do have side effects, like bloating, gas, and diarrhea. Regardless of what calorie route you take, YOU HAVE TO SENSIBLY EXERCISE to increase "bodily tone" and calorie expenditure. Most foods carry calorie information and most exercise machines will calculate your calorie expenditures. A little extra reading will answer your questions; you have to become committed.

    THERE IS NOTHING THAT SUCCEEDS LIKE SUCCESS. If you set unrealistic goals, you're bound to fall short and give up. DON'T SHOOT FOR THE MOON. Settle for slow, but steady progress; like 1-2 pound weight loss per week. Don't hang around bars, buffets and finger-food events. Why put yourself in situations that make it harder to say no? Similarly, if you are a junk food junkie, you'll have to make a determined, conscious effort to wean yourself away from that lifestyle. Be honest with yourself. You're the only one that will make the ultimate difference. Help is there for the asking.

Be very careful with ads promoting procedures, devices and pharmaceuticals. "Fat burning pills" are usually uppers, or useless. Uppers are like putting high-octane gas in a lawnmower. Sooner or later the engine burns out. Anything touted to boost your metabolism has to be viewed with suspicion. Ask, what are the scientific studies? Verify by contacting the FDA and your state boards of pharmacy and medicine.

"Lipo-dissolves, liposuction, lap-band procedures, surgical stapling and/or gastric bypass... ALL have serious potential for unwanted side effects. Some products and procedures are approved by the FDA and the medical community, other are not. YOU HAVE TO DO THE RESEARCH AND UNDERSTAND THE RISKS VERSUS THE BENEFITS. <u>GET EVERYTHING IN WRITING.</u>

The Las Vegas Review Journal, January 4, 2005, reported on an article in the Annals of Internal Medicine.

"A review of 10 of the nation's most popular weight-loss programs found that except for Weight Watchers, none of them offer proof that they actually work at helping people shed pounds", <u>and keep them off.</u> Other programs may be effective (short term or long term) but good documentation is lacking, despite claims from those pushing their special interests.

The article went on to say, "About 45 million Americans diet each year. People in this country spend $1 billion to $2 billion per year on weight-loss programs. But millions of those who enroll in weight-loss programs every year do not have much to go on when choosing a diet plan because few studies have been done that pass scientific muster."

Don't be misled by labels that proclaim, "No cholesterol, all natural and loaded with healthful antioxidants". Look at the calorie content and match it to your metabolic bank account.

We're continuously bombarded with promos for 'total body' diagnostic scans, blood tests, ultrasound probes and other high tech promises for discovering defects. The golden rule in medicine has been, and continues to be, **NOTHING SUBSTITUTES FOR A GOOD HISTORY AND PHYSICAL EXAMINATION.**

Reality is that tests make money, are often not necessary and may lead to unwanted/unintended consequences. However, since many people are programmed to think tests are the end-all for everything, health care providers are quick to order tests first, running up the costs next and thinking last. It's a well-accepted medical teaching that a detailed history and careful medical exam, by a well-trained physician, will make the diagnosis (or come close to it) 90 percent of the time. It might take the better part of an hour for a first time visit….not welcomed by managed care, bottom line pencil pushers. There is no justification to order tests first and talk to the patient second. Tests are there to confirm tentative diagnoses, develop a diagnoses not derived from doing a history and physical and/or to follow the patient's progress with therapeutic intervention.

Direct marketing, internet access and media hype have, in my opinion, compounded problems of healthcare delivery. The people behind these promotions frequently give half-truths, misinformation and promises from fantasia. Consider this scenario:

A 60-year old female, admitted prior smoker, overweight with elevated blood pressure, is worried about having coronary artery disease. She's seen the ads and read the promos for diagnostic angiography. She tells her doctor she wants an angiogram. Do you think it should be done?

My answer is maybe, but very likely not. She does have cardiac risk factors, but no signs or symptoms of cadiovascular disease. I would run other lab tests to document lipid levels (cholesterol profile and triglycerides), fasting blood sugar, c-reactive protein and A1c level to assess sugar metabolism, do a stress EKG (non-invasive), lay out a weight loss/exercise program and set goals for blood pressure reduction with appropriate medications and weight reduction.

Angiography, an invasive procedure, does carry risks of bleeding, artery blockage, irregular heart rhythms, heart damage and/or death. In skilled hands the risk is small but if it happens to you it's 100 percent. There has to be appropriate hard data to justify invasive procedures.

The doctor should explain the risks of invasive procedures and discuss whether she is prepared to change her lifestyle if significant cardiovascular disease is uncovered?

Will she go on a diet, exercise, do whatever it takes to control blood pressure and continue to refrain from smoking? If the angiographic findings are serious enough, is she prepared to accept angioplasty (dilating the artery and possibly using a stent) or open heart surgery? There may be other, less invasive tests to try first, like intravenous nuclear imaging. There again, all risks and limitations of proposed tests have to be discussed with the patient and adequately documented. It takes time to counsel such a patient. Counseling does not pay as well as doing tests and procedures. Even well-intentioned doctors may be pressed into taking the easier, higher paying route...especially with a patient pressuring the doctor because of advertising promos, and costs being picked up by third party payers and not the patient. The easy route may not be the best route. I'll discuss another case under STRESS EKG's (exercise stress electrocardiograms).

Communication and documentation is extremely important. Here are a few points I saw discussed in a Southwest Airline's Spirit Magazine.

    a. Have a family doctor who knows you, your family and your history.
    b. Make a list of what you'd like to discuss at your next visit.
    c. Bring up the most important things first.
    d. Don't take internet information as absolute truth.
    e. Be assertive in getting satisfactory answers. The atmosphere should be mutually comfortable.
    f. If you don't understand, ask again or bring someone along who might help.
    g. Discuss everything: medicines you're on, religious beliefs as it effects care, family

histories, important feelings, alternative healthcare, lifestyles, habits, risks versus benefits, any changes in mood and bodily functions.

h. If your healthcare provider doesn't have time to listen and talk, find one that will.

ANNUAL SCREENING FOR WOMEN

1. Establish a good working relationship with a primary care physician. Check out the doctor's credentials (Google, the County and State Medical Societies). You can ask for references, (especially when considering elective surgical procedures), availability, coverage when the doctor is not around and communication skills. Does your doctor have the 4A's?

   AVAILABILITY?
   AFFORDABILITY?
   ACCESSIBILITY
   AFFABILITY?

2. Visit the doctor anytime you notice a change in how you feel and/or how you function. Get in the habit of an annual, preventive checkup. This should not be overly costly, complicated or time consuming. It should start with an updated history and complete physical

examination. Basic laboratory tests are: CBC (complete blood count), urine analysis (simple dip stick), chemistries that check a thyroid panel, lipids (cholesterol and tryiglycerides), kidney function (creatinine and BUN), liver function panel, fasting blood sugar and A1c level. Other lab tests may be indicated if you are on medications that require specific monitoring, or to follow-up findings in the history and/or physical exam.

A baseline resting EKG and a front and side view chest x-ray should be done on the initial visit, and then once every five years.... unless signs and symptoms suggest repeat investigations. A baseline pap smear starting around age 12 (maybe later, depending on your doctor's knowledge of your family history and family lifestyles), and then every three years... again, depending on your personal situation.

3. With normal risk patients, I would encourage breast self- examination one to two years after puberty. A baseline mammogram at around age 18 and then every two years. Baseline means getting the test while you're in good health, with no complaints (signs or symptoms). Women at high risk for breast cancer should be

checked more frequently by themselves, and by their physician. With a strong family history of cancer you may want to know what genetic testing is available and what options go with positive testing. Don't do testing for the sake of testing. You have to have very specific reasons to test, with a clear plan for follow-up.
4. In people who do not have risk factors for bowel cancer, exam by colonoscopy (or a procto-sigmoidoscopy with a double contrast barium enema) can be done once for baseline data, at age 35-40, and then once every 10 years. Baseline data goes into your records and can be used for comparison at later dates.

I've seen patients who had been advised to have surgery for suspicious "spot(s)" on a chest x-ray. By looking at old x-rays it was determined the "spot (s)" in question had been around for years, had not changed and was not significant. Not every doctor takes the time to enquire about and/or retrieve old records and x-rays. This is not an acceptable medical practice. It should be routinely done.

5. A relatively newer procedure for bowel examination is called virtual colonoscopy. It requires the swallowing of a miniature

camera and carries no reported risks. It's still being evaluated and may not be covered by most insurance plans. CAT scans, MRI's, whole body imaging, ultrasonography, stress EKG's, Holter Monitors and the like are only justified after a complete history and physical exam (documented), routine lab and x-ray……then use specialized procedures and equipment as professionally needed to make a diagnosis and/or to follow therapeutic intervention.

ANNUAL SCREENING FOR MEN

1. Find a physician, as described for women, and get baseline and annual exams.
2. Men, as with women, should get into the same routine of having yearly preventive medical visits with baseline laboratory and imaging exams. There are a few differences, other than where men and women may come from (Venus or Mars). Men have testicles and prostates; women have ovaries and vaginas….I hope this is no revelation to the reader.
3. Men can get breast cancer and/or harmless breast enlargements. Check

with a good generalist or endocrinologist (specialist in glands and hormones) if male breast enlargement arises. The testicles should always be examined on a *routine* male physical examination.

4. The prostate is easily examined with the doctor's finger and a blood test (PSA). In my opinion, ultrasound is NOT justified unless a digital (finger) exam and a blood test (PSA) has raised concerns about the status of the prostate. Biopsy of the prostate is similarly not justified until the aforementioned exams and tests have been done. There are medically acceptable options if prostatic cancer has been diagnosed. The most important point to remember: THERE IS NO IMMEDIATE RUSH. You have plenty of time to get other opinions about hormone therapy, no therapy, external beam radiation, radiation seeds or surgery. Your choice depends on many factors. Your urologist, radiotherapist and/or surgeon should carefully explain the pros and cons for your informed consideration. You not only need to know the efficacy and indications for the various options, you need to know the side effects of your choices. Screening for prostate cancer should start around age 40.

Now for a few pet peeves; applicable for both men and women:

LUNG CANCER

I have rarely seen a primary lung cancer (one starting in the lung) in a person who did not smoke. It happens, but in my experience, not often. Regardless of all the x-rays, CAT scans or MRI's, once the diagnosis has been made, the overall 5-year survival rate (2009) is roughly 10 percent. In other words, early detection methods are lousy, as is effective treatment for cures. **DON'T SMOKE,** and if you do, **QUIT**. As for second hand smoke, exposure to the smoke of others, I originally thought claims were overblown. However, I think the evidence is currently quite convincing that second hand smoke does carry an increased risk for lung cancer.

In Nevada, one out of four women smoke; the highest percentage of female smokers in the country. Will it change? Ask the promoters, the lobbyists and the legislators. Nevada is also at or near the top for lung cancer, and head and neck cancer. It has nothing to do with atomic testing or air quality. It has to do with smoking and drinking, which incidentally are gaming's fellow travelers.

Nevada's major industry is not interested in seriously changing those habits. Spend a few hours in our older casinos and you'll have to hang your clothes outside to dissipate the ashtray odor. The newer casinos are supposed to have better air filtration systems…I could name a few that smell no better than the older establishments. A few places tried to be smoke-free casinos. They didn't last too long. If you're in denial about your odds for winning in a casino, you might as well be consistent in denying your odds for lung cancer when you smoke? At least don't do it around kids.

SCREENING FOR BOWEL CANCER

Early detection methods are lousy. Screening for blood in the stool usually leads to frustration; patient compliance for sample collection is very poor and such testing rarely finds cancer. Maybe the test in which you add a chemical into the toilet bowel will be more acceptable than tests requiring retrievable of a stool sample by the patient; i.e. actually transferring a sample of stool onto material for testing. My experiences and observations indicate that getting a positive test for blood in the stool rarely leads to a diagnosis of cancer. The positive finding was usually the result of insignificant bleeding from rectal irritation and/or minor tears (fissures). Those in low risk categories (negative family histories) could use a baseline colon exam around age 35-40, and then every 10 years. Higher risk persons should start around age 30 and be examined more frequently. No matter what you do, early detection of bowel cancer is very difficult and treatment options are limited. Many times the discovery is purely fortuitous. Causes are unclear and most likely multifactorial. High fiber diets and aspirin have been shown NOT to influence the incidence of bowel cancer. Early detection, does provide a good chance for surgical cure. Stages III or IV (spread beyond the bowel wall) have very poor outlooks. In my opinion, colonoscopy, like ultrasound of the prostate, has been inappropriately done in too many patients; obviously for economic gain. Any physician can buy a scope or ultrasound setup and go "into business". Most get appropriate training and follow sound guidelines; too many don't.

One family practitioner took a 3-day course at Lake Tahoe. The colonoscope manufacturer sponsored the meeting and paid for travel, room, meals and ski tickets. The practitioner bought the equipment and did the scoping as an outpatient procedure in one of the lesser (in my opinion) Las Vegas hospitals. The practitioner got all excited when he thought he finally discovered something of significance on one of his colonoscopies; he saw a dark mass in the sigmoid area. He had the good presence to call a board certified colorectal surgeon for an immediate consult. The surgeon looked into the scope and determined the head of the scope had bent in a U-shaped fashion and the family practitioner was looking at himself, so to speak. Colonoscopy does carry the risk of bowel perforation and bleeding. I prefer a proctosigmoidoscopy with a double contrast barium enema as an initial screening exam.

STRESS ELECTROCARDIOGRAMS (EKG's)

This is where the patient is put on a treadmill, exercise bicycle, or other device to evaluate the heart's function while the patient exercises. Engineers have produced relatively compact units with diagnostic printouts. Although the technology is good, nothing is perfect. Errors do occur with machines and/or humans. Any physician can buy a machine, as with scopes and ultrasound equipment, and unleash a cash cow. Equipment manufacturers are like lobbyists; they wine, dine and do whatever it takes to sell their wares. It's relatively easy for the practitioner to enter statements into the record to justify his doing a stress EKG, and have an insurer pay the bill. What harm, other than monetary, you ask? Consider this scenario:

A healthy, 35-year old fireman reports for his annual physical examination. He has no family history of heart disease. He has no signs or symptoms of heart or circulatory problems. He has no risk factors: non-smoker, no diabetes, not overweight, normal blood pressure, good exercise habits and good blood cholesterol and triglyceride levels. He also has a normal, resting electrocardiogram. He read in a magazine that it would be "good" to have an annual stress EKG as part of a yearly check-up. He wasn't told about false positives or false negatives. His insurance did cover stress EKG's so the fireman decided to ask for the "freebie" and his physician complied with the fireman's request.

If the stress EKG comes up with a false negative interpretation (which can happen in the best of hands) i.e. he's told that everything is okay when actually the test missed identifying coronary artery disease, sooner or later his disease will become apparent. However, if the test suggests coronary disease (a positive), then further testing has to be done. False positives also occur in the best of hands; i.e. the test is read as showing disease when it is later determined there was no disease. The doctor told the fireman:

"Looks like you may have problems with circulation to your heart. We can do an isotope scan. We inject radioactive contrast material into a vein while you exercise and view your heart's function on a TV-like monitor. There is no risk to the procedure. We'll test you for sensitivity to the contrast material."

The fireman agrees and the test is done. The doctor now says:

"Unfortunately the radioactive scan did not give us a definitive answer. We should go on and do the "gold standard" test...angiography. We put a plastic tube into an artery in your groin and feed it up into the beginning of your coronary circulation. We then inject dye (contrast material) and watch it flow through your heart circulation. We'll test you for sensitivity to the contrast material."

The physician might have skipped the isotope scan and recommended going directly to an angiogram (as some do). This patient is now somewhat weary and leery with testing.

"You know, doc, this angiogram stuff sounds a little scary."

"Not really," replies his doctor. "We've done it thousands of times. It not only allows us to actually see if you have significant blockage to any of your coronary arteries, it also gives us a chance to correct serious findings by using a balloon to open the blockage and use a stint to keep it open."

What the doctor may fail to tell him, or glibly gloss over, is the fact that serious complications occur at an average rate of 1 per 3000 angiographies…even in the best of hands. The complications can be perforation of an artery, irritation of the lining of an artery causing complete blockage, rhythm disturbances or combinations thereof. Because of these complicating possibilities, which may become life-threatening, all angiographic procedures are supposed to have surgical backup teams available for immediate intervention should the need arise. Remember, giving you statistical odds does not emphasize the reality that if it happens to you, it's 100 percent bad.

This is not a hypothetical scenario…it happened (and it continues to happen). This man had his angiogram which turned out to be 100 percent normal. He went home and complained about decreasing exercise tolerance. He was re-evaluated by another cardiologist who said he now had a resting EKG that showed changes from his pre-angiogram tracings; i.e. the current EKG suggested circulation problems to his heart. He agreed to another angiogram which showed that the first procedure must have irritated the lining of his right coronary artery. This caused a clot and permanent blockage of the artery. We now had a 35-year old man who came in for a routine annual checkup and was taken down the slippery slope of un-justified cardiac tests (no history, no signs or symptoms, no adverse lifestyle for coronary artery disease). His normal heart was now minus 1/3 of his original circulation. I, and the second cardiologist, offered to testify (at no charge) if he initiated a malpractice suit. His records clearly indicated he was not given information about the risks of his procedures, which were done without medical justification. He did not sue; which puzzles me to this day.

THE MAJOR POINT IS: YOU DON'T DO TESTS (ESPECIALLY INVASIVE TESTS THAT CARRY SIGNIFICANT RISKS) JUST BECAUSE THE TESTS ARE AVAILABLE AND SOMEONE ELSE WILL PAY FOR IT. A VALID MEDICAL INDICATION AND/OR NECESSITY HAS TO EXIST.

A word about heart risk factors. This is important when evaluating worker's compensation cases. The American Heart Association lists five major risk factors: family history, smoking, high blood pressure, diabetes and abnormal lipid levels (blood fats). Stress and overweight may be contributing factors by affecting eating habits and exercise, which in turn worsen the Heart Association's five risk factors. Interesting debates arise about what actually constitutes chronic stress. Consensus, in my opinion, has not emerged. Acute stress, however, can precipitate a heart attack.... you exceed the circulatory capacity to supply blood and oxygen to a diseased system. We do have visitors come to the desert, party all night and go play tennis in 110 degrees the next day. These overweight, diabetic, hypertensive, heavy-smoking jocks are physically stressing their systems....rolling the dice in the casino, partying and carrying on at the tennis courts; not a good idea for those with medically high risk profiles.

THE PATIENT IS NOT JUST NUMBERS

Some physicians over-react to laboratory numbers. I've seen patients with high total cholesterols as their <u>only</u> cardiac risk factor. You can try diet modification and adding a statin-type drug, but I see no sense in driving the person crazy by becoming obsessed with attaining a given number. If you can reasonably achieve what are currently accepted goals in medical circles, fine. If not, leave the patient alone. The majority will do very well.....in my opinion. Sometimes the best medicine is to sit on your hands and do nothing.

BONE DENSITY

To me, this is a good example of technology creating an industry...a very lucrative industry for equipment manufacturers, drug developers and entrepreneurial healthcare personnel. It sounds like a broken record, but any well-trained physician should be able to spot the at-risk fracture patient with the history and physical exam. It's your elderly, frail-looking female, who usually eats poorly and never exercises. Remember the saying, "if you don use it, you lose it." Exercise is important to bone integrity.

It doesn't take a genius to realize that an older, relatively inactive person, with possibly poor vision, unsteady gait and questionable dietary habits is more prone to slip, trip or fall and break one or more bones. I don't need a bone density to verify the risk. From my experiences, there is no question that bone density tests are grossly over-ordered, and many times mis-reported. I've had patients tested for bone density as a routine. Some were told their bones were "not good". They asked me about suggested medication. I advised many of them to tell the physician making the referral and/or bone density tester that they will take the prescribed medication...but actually not take it, and have the test repeated 3-6 months later.

Surprise, the repeat test is read as "improved bone density". Wow, how's that for a placebo effect? It helped the patient get a better report, and the person doing the bone density test got more revenue.

If you do consider a patient at risk for a bone fracture, as described above, what medications would you recommend? They all carry significant caveats: Fosamax and Evista may interfere with other medications. Read the package inserts; diarrhea or other gastrointestinal irritation may occur. Remember what I said in the chapter on drug safety. Don't be too eager to jump on the new-medication bandwagon. Wait a few years and see what happens after the drug has come on to the market. Look at female hormone replacement, for example. After many years of putting hundreds of thousands of women on female hormones, we finally got the data indicating that doing so put some at higher risk for heart disease and/or cancer. Hot flashes and flushes can be treated with safer methods.

COSMETIC SURGERY

I'm surprised no one has come up with a Las Vegas make-over package deal (at least I'm not aware of any): airfare, lodging, gaming chips, meals…all inclusive package for your fantasy make-over. I'm not talking about reconstructive surgeries for birth defects, trauma or post-cancer treatment. I'm referring to elective cosmetic surgery. It's over-done and under regulated…in my opinion. I see too many procedures being done without adequate evaluation of the patient's motives, expectations and understandings. Hustlers take advantage of human vulnerabilities. It's up to our legislators to enact laws making medical providers meaningfully liable for inappropriate acts.

A word about the changing world of adult vaccines: as of 2008:

- I would strongly recommend annual flu shots for people with general medical and/or lung problems.
- I would strongly recommend Shingles (Herpes Zoster) vaccine for seniors over age 60; even those who've had Shingles.
- I would strongly recommend Gardisil (Human Papilloma Vaccine, HPV) for all females ages 8 to 35. This could well be extended to age 50, and to males in the coming years. HPV not only causes female cervical cancer; it has been linked to other female genital tract cancers, rectal cancers and various head and neck cancers.

- **Booster shots and travel protection data are readily available to your physician and yourself through your county and state health departments and/or federal Centers for Disease Control and Prevention (CDC).**

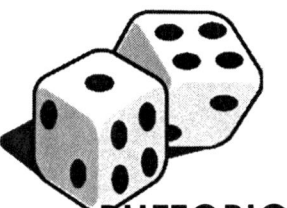

CHAPTER VII

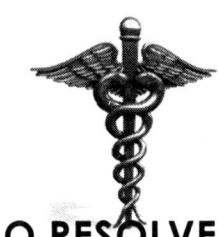

RHETORIC AND PANDERING, NO RESOLVE

Politicians proclaim positions that strike the right chords. Hypocrisy, pandering and promises of simple solutions get them elected. Once elected, the solutions appear to get complicated and pre-election promises evaporate. Universal healthcare, single payer plans, medical malpractice reform, overhaul of the pharmaceutical industry and the FDA, reigning in healthcare costs and balancing the budget are standard political refrains emanating from both sides of the political aisle. If I were in charge, I know what I'd do and how I would do it. Don't get enthused, or alarmed. I am not a candidate for higher office and I see no ground swell to draft me as a candidate.

Let's start with the important topic of medical malpractice. It's been around since the beginning of humankind, like original sin. If you think ethical, professional and moral concerns weren't evident early on, why did Hippocrates feel the need to create his oath? He obviously realized all men were not created morally or ethically equal, nor did they universally learn to respond with the highest thoughts and actions. Scientific breakthroughs, like stem cell research, cloning, genetic counseling, organ transplants and life support decisions have raised additional opportunities to bend the rules of reason. Trial lawyers love controversy; it keeps them in business. Here are some interesting national statistics, from National Practitioner Data Bank (NPDB) and Jury/Verdict Research.

LIABILITY COSTS

- Adds 60-180 billion to the cost of healthcare annually.
- National median awards doubled between 1995 and 2000.
- Settlement values increased 16% between 1995 and 2000.

MEDIAN VERDICTS

- Childbirth $ 2,050,000
- Misdiagnosis-cancer $ 1,000,000
- Treatment delay $ 1,000,000
- Misdiagnosis-other $ 750,000
- Medication error $ 668,000
- Lack of informed consent $ 500,000
- Non-surgical treatment $ 400,688
- Surgical negligence $ 355,000

There's been a predictable change in the way medical practitioners behave. It's called DEFENSIVE MEDICINE. 59 percent of physicians believe that the fear of liability discourages open discussion and thinking about ways to reduce healthcare costs. 76 percent of physicians believe that litigation concerns have negatively impacted their ability to provide better quality health care.

Doctors will order more tests and call in more consultants to CYA…..cover their rears. More is not synonymous with increased quality of care, and it does drive up the costs of practicing medicine. Others will limit their practices so as to avoid high-risk patients and/or situations. Other practitioners will sour the important doctor/patient relationship by asking the patient to sign all kinds of disclaimers. It's akin to signing a prenuptial agreement. In my mind this does not project mutual trust.

A Las Vegas, board certified plastic and cosmetic surgeon has written a handbook, after 25 years in the profession. It was written as a teaching resource for the reconstructive surgeon. With his permission, I quote from his book, The Cosmetic Surgeon and the Law, by Dr. William H. Canada M.D.

"I have been practicing plastic and cosmetic surgery for many years. In all of that time, I have found this to be a very stressful profession. In my early years of practice, I imagined the stress would decrease as I became more knowledgeable and adept as a surgeon. This has not proven to be true. Each year the stress has increased rather decreased, based upon the escalation of the demands of insurance companies, the federal government and the medical-legal jurisprudence system.

It is not within my abilities to make these problems disappear. However, I do believe that if the information presented in this book is incorporated into your practice, it will make you more comfortable in responding to the accusation of malpractice."

The doctor goes on to cover such topics as advertising, dishonest practice policies, informed consent, giving a deposition, loose talk, good patient communication, sexual misconduct, going to trial, having a conservative approach to patient selection and in many instances, just plain common sense. The author-surgeon further stated:

"Statistics report that the average cosmetic surgeon will be sued once every three years. Since the usual time from the initiation of a suit to the time it takes to go to trial, takes three years, most plastic surgeons could just be finishing up one suit when another one presents itself.

Cosmetic surgery holds a unique distinction among surgical specialties. When a cosmetic surgeon accepts a patient for an operation, he is undertaking one of the most responsible tasks in surgery. He is performing surgery not to remove pathology, not to mend a defect, but to make that part of the body more beautiful. Contrary to other fields of surgery, your work is on display to many people. All have an opinion on the quality of your work, whether that opinion is correct or not. Complete strangers can be the initiating factor in causing your patient to become dissatisfied and to become litigious. The husband of the recent breast augmentation patient says he doesn't like your patient's new breasts. This certainly can turn a formerly happy breast enlargement patient into one who is decidedly dissatisfied. Then there is the mother-in-law who doesn't like her daughter-in-law's new nose. If the truth were known, that mother-in-law doesn't like anything about the daughter-in-law, past or present."

Dr. Canada is refreshingly frank in his Chapter 3 entitled, DISHONEST PRACTICE POLICIES. He zeros in on patient complicity and physician compliance. There is no question doctor's have to do a better job of policing their own! Let's start by having the remaining 13 states adopt the policy of a single board for the licensing of DO's and MD's. As of 2008, 37 states do just that.

Ethics reform includes lawyers, corporate executives, lobbyists, legislators and the population at large. Continuing with Dr. Canada's candid assessments:

"In any community that has two or more cosmetic surgeons, there is invariably a dishonest apple in the barrel. This is the type of surgeon who lies about the patient's diagnosis in order to have the surgery paid by an insurance company. (i.e. doing a rhinoplasty and calling it surgery for deviated a septum, rather than calling it a rhinoplasty for a cosmetic change.) The deviated septum did not exist but insurance doesn't cover elective cosmetic procedures.

This dishonesty makes the crooked surgeon very competitive in relation to his colleagues who are truthful about the preoperative diagnosis. If the dishonest surgeon also has his own private operating facility, then it's almost impossible to prove his falsifications.

Without question, you know your own colleagues who are dishonest in your area. (As an example): on the surgery schedule, the surgery to be performed is listed as a breast biopsy. However, you see him going into the surgical suite with a pair of breast implants under his arm.

Other examples of pervasive practices: The cosmetic surgeon who has never seen a nose that did not need a septoplasty or submucous resection. Listing the patient with small, ptotic breasts as a reduction mammoplasty. The abdominoplasty with doubtful hernias or diastasis (separation) of the rectus abdominus muscles. The ophthalmologist who only does upper eyelid blepharoplasty (he can fudge the field of vision test and get insurance to pay for what is really cosmetic surgery).

While I am well aware that the perpetrators of these frauds are rarely caught or disciplined, they are caught occasionally, and with more frequency as State Boards of Medicine become more aggressive. (Certainly not true, in my opinion, in the state of Nevada).

When the dishonest surgeon falsifies the preoperative diagnosis, the patient is usually aware that it is happening. Now if the surgery that was not listed correctly is in the operative and/or insurance report, and the result has major complications that results in a malpractice suit, the offending surgeon is in a very difficult situation. If the plaintiff's attorney can prove that the surgeon lied about the surgery that was performed, the jury is not about to believe anything else the surgeon has to say.

A vindictive patient may also report the surgeon's dishonesty to the State Board of Medicine. This could result in the surgeon losing his medical license. My advice is to be scrupulously honest in all your business activities. When patients have actually asked me to falsify an insurance report, my standard reply has been; a physician who falsifies your records is dishonest. If they are dishonest with an insurance company, do you think they would not be dishonest with you? Do you really want a crook doing surgery on you or your family?

Another example of dishonest practice policies is patient solicitation.

The following happened in Las Vegas. A Beverly Hills plastic surgeon flew into Las Vegas every weekend to do cosmetic surgery. He had hired a fulltime nurse who actively solicited for breast augmentation in all the topless bars in town. She actually took a portfolio of his before and after photos, and gave mini-lectures to her topless clients on the fabulous abilities of her employer. She also informed her prospective clients that her plastic surgeon had invented a new way of doing breast enlargement surgery that was superior to any other technique in the country."

Dr. Canada listed the legal minefields created by the Beverly Hill's plastic surgeon.

1. **PATIENT ABANDONEMENT:** The nurse followed the patient after surgery until the surgeon returned from Los Angeles one week later.
2. **FRAUD:** He professed to have a special technique for doing the surgery. It was not special or original.
3. **SOLICITATION**: In many states a violation of prohibited solicitation or drumming, is classified as a Class A misdemeanor."

Patients have the responsibility of being honest and making it clear to your health providers, that you want them to follow the rules. You have to get after the legislators to insure unequivocal laws for ethical healthcare delivery, with severe penalties for transgressors…and you have be a whistleblower when the rules are not followed.

This is a national problem. Look in the yellow pages of the phone book. Read local newspaper and TV ads. We have a national epidemic of healthcare providers pitching hair restoration, liposuction, lipo-dissolve, diet surgery, hormone therapy, rejuvenation schemes—you name it. Healthcare providers pitch it and consumers catch it…especially if they can get third party payers to cover it.

The Las Vegas Review Journal carried a commentary by writer Jane Ann Morrison, in October 2003. It discussed the sexual relationship of an Osteopathic doctor, with two of his patients. This doctor was also accused of using animal grade Botox for cosmetic injections. The accusations were proved accurate in courts of law. The man is still practicing medicine. The doctor's lawyer didn't think it was a big deal for any professional to sleep with his patients. Jane Ann Morrison quoted the lawyer as saying:

"This is a fact pattern that repeats itself in every profession, whether a journalist or a lawyer; it's not a case where a doctor took advantage of someone."

The lawyer claimed it was consensual but the courts didn't buy it. Do 'fact patterns' make it ethical/legal? The phrase, "fact pattern", is a new twist for me, and using animal grade Botox falls under the Latin phrase, Res Ipse Loquitor; The Thing Speaks For Itself."

The Government Accounting Office several years ago estimated an annual loss of over 15 billion dollars due to fraud and abuse of the Medicare/Medicaid program. It then went to 30 to 50 billion a year. It is now (2008) estimated to be over 100 billion. I don't see legislators rushing to make corrections.

I consider the southern Nevada medical community fortunate in having a colleague with an MD and JD degree; Dr. Weldon (Don) Havins. He is a Board Certified Ophthalmologist who has acted as CEO, and Special Counsel and President of the Clark County Medical Society. He had a nice discussion, in the December 2002 issue of the COUNTY LINE newsletter, of ETHICS AND TRUTH IN MEDICINE AND LAW, drawing attention to similarities and diversities. His summary is applicable to forming an opinion about physicians having sexual liaisons with a patient...consensual or not.

"The medical and legal professions generally agree on what the ethical principles are (e.g. beneficence, integrity, justice), and that they ought to comply with them. The professions have distinctive different theories on the methods of discovering the truth or facts. The professions differ markedly on the ethics of fee-splitting, contingency fees and a sexual relationship with a client/patient. The effect and significance of professional malpractice differs profoundly."

Dr. Havins goes on to say, "Respected law professor, Richard Wasserstrom, posits that in contrast to the physicians' scientific methodology, the adversarial (legal) system encourages the lawyer to be: competitive rather than cooperative, aggressive rather than accommodating, ruthless rather than compassionate and pragmatic rather than principled." Dr. Havins then asks:

"Are the ethics of one professional more than the other? Or are the founding principles and traditions of the respective Codes just different?"

There's a lot to think about.

When the topic of ethics is brought up, a physician will usually think of the Hippocratic Oath, and then possibly the American Medical Association's (AMA's) Code of Ethics. A big question is why, in 2003, only 29 percent of the nation's one million physicians belonged to the AMA? In 1972, 75 percent were members of the AMA. In my opinion, most physician non-members feel the AMA has not effectively acted on their behalf.

I went sour on the AMA in the 1980's when it was obvious the leadership was not following its own code and rhetoric. The long-standing AMA Executive Director, Dr. Sammons MD, was among other things, exposed for providing interest-free AMA loans to "buddies". It was also revealed that he was receiving an annual salary in excess of half a million dollars, plus perks. I asked for a written disclosure of all other administrative salaries. I was refused that information even though I had been an AMA member since 1960. I asked the Clark County Medical Society (as a member of the Executive Board) to protest the non-disclosure of the AMA's administrative salaries. They weren't interested. Happily, the Society has become more administratively and politically engaged in the 21st Century. Despite the improvement, I have to chuckle at a friend's (a mining engineer) characterization of doctor's in politics:

"They're like virgins in a whore house. They're not sure why they're there, and they can't wait to leave."

As for the AMA, it originally appeared to me to have a centrist position, regardless of political party affiliation. Today, many of us perceive it as being far to the left, and aligned more often than not with wealthy personal injury lawyers. Take, for example, the AMA's joining a group of personal injury lawyer's class action lawsuit in Miami, against the nation's eight largest health insurers. While doctors may have problems with those insurers, they are still the primary payers for many of the their patients. You don't make deals with the devil (trial lawyers) in an attempt to solve short-term problems with a third party payer;

deal directly with the third party. When the class-action is completed, the lawyers will walk off with 40-50 percent of the spoils. What will the doctor's get?

Or, take the AMA's championing a patient's bill of rights. Talk about ignoring *unintended consequences*. This sound-good rhetoric, in reality, gives lawyers *foundations* from which to formulate tort cases. I remember the old saying from my Army days…never volunteer.

On the subject of tort reform, Dr. Charles Krauthammer MD wrote in TIME magazine, January 13, 2003:

"Surgeons in West Virginia have gone on strike to protest the exorbitant cost of malpractice insurance; good for them. Don't talk to me about the ethics of doctor's going on strike. So long as they agree to treat emergency cases, they have as much right to strike as anyone else. The premise of a free market is that people can withhold their labor if they find the conditions under which they work intolerable.

Many doctors do. Many, especially those in the inherently risky specialties such as surgery, and obstetrics (anesthesia, neurosurgery and emergency/trauma), have been forced out of business by malpractice premiums or hounded out by malpractice litigation. A totally irresponsible legal system, driven by a small cadre of lawyers who have hit the mother lode, has produced perhaps the most dysfunctional medical-liability system in the world. Juries hand out millions of dollars not just for lost earnings but also in capricious punitive damages in which the number of zeros attached to the penalty seems to be chosen at random.

As a result, innocent doctors who have devoted their lives to their patients are required to spend tens, even hundreds, of thousands of dollars a year on insurance. In effect, we are making doctors give up an entire chunk of each year's laboring just to work off their insurance premiums. Why? To cover for the few offenders in their midst: to compensate the lucky few victims who stumble upon the most profligate juries: and most important, to make a few trial lawyers very, very rich. (Dr. Krauthammer is no longer in practice).

This is not a hard problem to fix. Tort reform is not rocket science. A reasonable bill passed the national House of Representatives in 2002 but died in the Senate, where the trial-lawyer lobby rules (sadly, Democrats, who historically championed worker's benefits, helped kill the reform package). The elements of a fix are simple; no limits on plaintiff's lost earnings or other costs, a reasonable cap on pain and suffering (non-economic damages--$250,000 in the House bill), a similar cap on punitive damages and serious penalties for frivolous lawsuits. Sliding fee scales for trial lawyers are also appropriate.

Of course there will be medical errors, and there will be medical malefactors. The bad doctors need to be found, punished and defrocked. But why should their sins be paid for by the good doctors among them? (called *unjust collective punishment*).

The current system is crazy, ruinous and unfair. It is easily changed: by lawyers."

Dr. Ann S. Lofsky, M.D. gave an excellent presentation on "THE MEDICAL MALPRACTICE CRISES" for the New Horizons medical meeting, Steamboat Springs, Colorado, February 7, 2007. Here is some of her data:

California enacted medical malpractice reform legislation in 1973-74, called MICRA, with four major components. They have stood the test of time and judicial scrutiny.

1. Mandated a $250,000 cap on non-economic damages ONLY (pain and suffering). No cap for treatment, lost wages, etc.

2. **Allows introduction into evidence of collateral sources of payment. There is no justification to having two or more sources pay for the same damages. Assign responsibility and have the allowed damages paid once.**
3. **Allow periodic payments of future damages (as opposed to mandatory lump-sum payments).**
4. **Provided for a sliding scale limit on attorney's contingency fees. Which, in effect gives up to 17% more of a settlement to the patient...not the lawyer.**

The Doctor's Company (1976–2004) reported that MICRA helped reduce California's medical liability premium rates by 33 %. The same company reported malpractice reform in Colorado (1986–2002) reduced Colorado liability premium rates 61%.

MICRA-type legislation has reduced verdict costs and frequency, <u>DIRECTLY INCREASED PATIENT'S BENFITS</u> (by invoking sliding scale limits on attorney's contingency fees), reduced average time to settlement and decreased costs of defensive medicine practices (Stanford Study showed states with effective tort reform had lower health care costs of 5-9%. Savings nationally could save $50 billion; Health and

Human Services estimated savings as high as $110 billion if reforms were adopted federally; i.e. in all states).

STATES WITH CAPS (2007)

- Colorado
- Florida
- Indiana
- Montana
- Texas
- Virginia
- Nevada (second vote pending)
- Georgia

- Idaho
- Mississippi
- South Carolina
- West Virginia
- Maryland
- Ohio

- Massachusetts
- Kansas

Dr. Lofsky summarized her presentation:
- We know, we do not speculate, real tort reform works.
- If society wishes to have astronomical indemnities, it must accept astronomical premiums, and astronomical healthcare costs.

Nevada's medical malpractice reform referendum passed in 2004. It will come up for a second vote in the next general election, before it can become permanent. KODIN (Keep Our Doctors in Nevada) coalition deserves credit for getting the proposal on the ballot and raising the money needed to educate the public and legislators…. and fight a nasty trial lawyer's coalition. It was the first time, in my experience, a significant number of Nevada physicians united and donated substantial money and time for much needed legislation. Three other states with similar referendums in 2004 failed in their attempts at medical malpractice reform. There is no excuse for not having federal legislators pass a MICRA-type package for every state in the union.

We really don't have to get academic, philosophic or cerebrally entangled when it comes to defining moral elements of fair play; i.e. good, functional patient/physician relationships. It comes down to living by THE GOLDEN RULE; doing unto others what you'd have them do unto you.

LIFE AND DEATH DECISIONS

Caregivers have to wrestle with questions about the quality of life, length of life and who decides. If an adult person has formulated definite wishes, should they become incapacitated, unconscious or faced with terminal illness, those wishes need to be documented and available when needed. It could avoid cases like Karen Quinlan and life support measures…or the more recent case of

Schaivo in Florida, focused on removal of feeding tubes. Parents, legal guardians or others are often required to make those very difficult decisions for non-adult persons. There are no hard and fast answers. You do the best you can with the cards you're dealt, and continually look toward better ways of doing it.

We get into all kinds of legalese when decisions have to be made on contraceptive advice about devises and supplies....especially with federally funded programs. Same applies to testing and treating sexually transmitted diseases, and screening and treating for illegal/controlled substance abuse.

Let's take an easy one, at least for me; legalizing marijuana for so-called medical use. I think it's totally uncalled for. I, as a physician, have an array of medications I can use to relieve the symptoms described by proponents for legalizing marijuana. In my professional opinion, **MARIJUANA HAS NO UNIQUE MEDICAL PROPERTIES OR ANY REDEEMING SOCIAL NEED!** I can give you a long list as to why marijuana is dangerous and unnecessary, and should remain illegal (contact me). We have enough problems with alcohol abuse. We don't need to add another drug to the mix.

We do not need opinions manufactured out of thin air. Extremist religious attitudes, special interests and biased-legal maneuverings do not foster constructive resolutions. I certainly don't have universal answers, but as a professional, I'm the one tasked with meeting the needs of society and the individual seeking medical help; I'm the one in the front line. We do have programs that work. Give us your input but allow us to do our job.

You want to ponder another headache? Consider access to medical care versus allocation of finite resources. Emergency rooms, intensive care units and military MASH facilities call it *TRIAGE*: i.e. take what you have, evaluate, sort and utilize your resources to help those most likely to benefit. The rest get what's left over. Judgement calls follow technical decisions; outcomes are never perfect. Try standing in the shoes of the primary responders before volunteering your opinions and thoughts.

What better way to end a chapter than paying tribute to a promising work in progress; a work I doubt many know about, and a work EVERYONE (lay and professional) could become part of. It's called

VIMI (VOLUNTEERS IN MEDICINE INSITTUTE)
www.vimi.org.

"Volunteers in Medicine is a proven, effective solution to the nation's number one problem, health care for the uninsured. The unique VIM model promotes a *CULTURE OF CARING*, while emphasizing the use of retired health care professionals and non-medical volunteers."

The idea is the brainchild of Dr. Jack B. McConnell, M.D., retired physician in Hilton Head, South Carolina, 1992. It's a story that fosters Goosebumps as you read the inscription in CIRCLE OF CARING, and the details of amazing volunteers on a selfless mission.

> "INSIDE EACH OF US IS A SENSE OF DECENCY
> AND GOODNESS AND IF WE LISTEN TO
> IT AND ACT
> ON IT, WE WILL GIVE THE WORLD
> MUCH OF THAT
> WHICH THE WORLD MOST NEEDS. IT IS NOT
> DIFFICULT BUT IT TAKES COURAGE TO LISTEN TO
> YOUR GOODNESS AND ACT ON IT."
> —Pablo Casals

As of December 2007, there are 61 Volunteers in Medicine Clinics across the country.

Alabama	–	Montgomery
California	–	El Cajon
Florida	–	Jacksonville, Lakeland, Port Charlotte, Stuart
Georgia	–	Brunswick, Dublin, Fayetteville, Jasper, Macon, Monroe, Savannah, Valdosta, Warner Robins
Indiana	–	Bloomington, Columbus, Indianapolis
Kansas	–	Manhattan
Louisiana	–	New Orleans
Massachusetts	–	Great Barrington
Mississippi	–	Oxford
Missouri	–	Hannibal, St. Charles
New Jersey	–	Cape May Court House, Pennsville, Red Bank
North Carolina	–	Brevard, Charlotte (2), Highlands, Jefferson, Laurinburg, Louisburg, Mathews, Mooresville, Raleigh, Supply
Ohio	–	Wooster
Oregon	–	Bend, Eugene
Pennsylvania	–	Berwick, Butler, Erie, Pittsburgh, Southampton State College, West Chester

South Carolina	–	**Aiken, Clinton, Hilton Head, Newberry, Taylors Woodruff**
Tennessee	–	**Chattanooga, Morristown, Tullahoma**
Texas	–	**McKinney**
Washington	–	**Port Angeles**
Wyoming	–	**Jackson**

VIM
162 St. Paul Street
Burlington, Vermont 05401

(802) 651-0112   www.vimi.org

Take the time to read about it. Tell your friends.

CHAPTER VIII

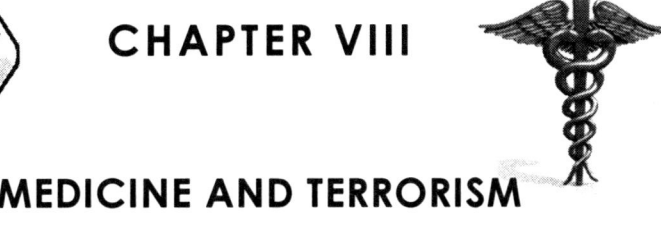

MEDICINE AND TERRORISM

With natural disasters like drought, earthquakes, volcanic eruptions, wildfires, storms and diseases, you'd think mankind would have enough to do without seeking better ways to kill each other. We've spent years going after smallpox and finally declaring it eradicated — only to have deranged minds attempt to resurrect it (and other infectious agents) for destructive purposes. How do you deal with these people and their regimes? They appear to be beyond logic and reason.

People bent on mischief, foreign or home grown, ecological deviants and political ideologues, can easily obtain knowledge and materials through libraries, on the internet and by watching TV. It's amazing we haven't had more incidents like 9/11. I think some of it is sheer luck.

Are we better prepared after 9/11? Perhaps slightly, but certainly not enough. As usually happens, well-intentioned funds all too often are diverted to self-interests and irrelevant projects. If you are not convinced get a copy of the hour long TV documentary, DUST TO DUST, a medical follow-up on the first responders and clean up crews at 9/11. State and federal authorities assured everyone the environmental mess posed no medical threat to the responders and bystanders. They didn't understand the risks of micronized cement dust, toxic metals, plastics and everything else in post 9/11 lower Manhattan. Among the countless costly blunders, they didn't issue appropriate self-contained respiratory equipment nor have they learned from their mistakes.

NUCLEAR

Nevada has had a long sanding relationship with the military, the government and nuclear R&D (research and development). We have Nellis Air Force Base, the Sandia run missile range at Tonopah, the Nevada Operations Office of the Department of Energy (DOE), the Department of Defense (DOD) and the Lawrence Livermore and Los Alamos National Laboratories. My direct observations and conclusions, as Medical Director of the Nevada Test Site operations for 18 years, are that no significant radiation exposures occurred as a result of above, or below ground atomic testing in Nevada. I'd be very happy to discuss, re-evaluate and look at data alleging otherwise. Similarly, no significant radiation exposures occurred form shipping, handling or storage of high level, partially spent nuclear materials from the United States <u>commercial</u> nuclear power industry—including theThree Mile Island incident. The same applies to our nuclear powered fleet. It's the safest technology this country has ever known.

Too bad this can't be said for the rest of the world. Russia is now our ally (at least on paper), but where are their scientists and nuclear materials? Russia's Vladimir Putin was interviewed on TV's 60 MINUTES before becoming President. He said his country could not account for all of their so-called suitcase nuclear devices. We know that Russian nuclear materials have been, and continue to be vulnerable to theft or unacceptable purchase? How many of their nuclear experts have relocated to new employers? The same applies to other nuclear powers with whom we do business, like India, Pakistan and China. The head of Pakistan's nuclear program is known to have sold vital technological information to unfriendly countries.

It is important to understand basic biologic and engineering facts in order to formulate valid opinions. Here are things you may not know.

There is a nice, wide, documentable margin of safety for exposure to ionizing radiation. If we didn't have this margin of safety, we wouldn't be able to use radiographic procedures for diagnostic dental and medical studies (x-rays, CAT scans and the like).

Ionizing radiation is a form of energy. Think of it like a fist hitting your body. We get a certain amount of normal hits every day from materials that make up our environment. The hits can be mild (as with alpha or beta radiation that doesn't, or minimally, penetrates the skin) or the hit can carry a big wallop if gamma radiation is involved.

Then there are factors like how many times you get hit over a given period of time, interval lengths for recovery, your individual susceptibility and other medical conditions. We don't need to go into the details. The important thing to remember is the wide margin of safety; i.e. we can take a lot of hits before sustaining irreversible damage.

The "Anti-" people make ridiculous statements like, "any exposure, no matter how small, causes significant damage…even if we can't measure or demonstrate it." It carries no scientific credibility. It amounts to playing speculative games with hypothetical, statistical numbers. Science fiction writers and entertainment media push their creative fantasies that lead to all sorts of misunderstandings and unnecessary fears (Jane Fonda and the movie China Syndrome, or Kiefer Sutherland and the TV series "24".)

We can scientifically demonstrate what radiation exposures are handled well by the body, what exposures lead to injury; some reversible, some not. We know what levels of tolerance exist for different organs and parts of the body. The lining of the bowel, for example, is very sensitive whereas bone is more resistant to radiation.

Another, very important but simple concept, is the distinction between exposure and contamination. If you stand in front of a radioactive source, like an x-ray machine, you get an exposure. It's a one-event occurrence, and how the body handles it, depends on the dose and type of radiation received (distance from the source and length of exposure figure into the calculations). You DO NOT become radioactive. Medical and dental diagnostic tests are designed to limit your exposure to safe levels. MRI's do not involve radiation (Magnetic Resonance Imaging), CAT scans do (Computerized Axial Tomography).

If there is a deliberate or accidental dispersion of radioactive materials (particles) like Iridium, Cesium or Plutonium, then you can be contaminated…internally and/or externally…. and the body has to be cleansed of the radioactive material.

It's all very simple….if you know what you're dealing with, and you are prepared to contain and/or treat it. I'm not convinced we've been doing all we should to be prepared. In Las Vegas, for example, the Oak Ridge National Laboratories (under DOE sponsorship), REACTS Program, puts on free periodic courses dealing with *Medical Response and Care of Radiation Accidents*. The program started around 1974. Aside from myself, there are just one or two physicians from the southern Nevada area who show up at these presentations. Most attendees are first responder fire department people. They are fairly knowledgeable, but what about the rest of "the team"; medical personnel, hospitals, etc.? With appropriate training, we could hope for a reasonable response to a bad event. Without training, it'll be chaos…like 9/11.

There are also voids in basic equipment. The fire department was discussing how it would handle an approach to an explosive incident (2007). I asked if their fire trucks had radiation detectors mounted on the front bumpers or windshields? It would be nice to know if your disaster included nuclear material. This is not a big-ticket item. The chief's response was:

"We've asked for it quite some time ago. It hasn't been supplied yet."

This is six years after 9/11 and God only knows how many billions of dollars allocated toward preparedness; no oversight, no accountability!

First responders have to know about the different types of radiation, their medical implications, whether they have exposure or contamination, what are the safe boundaries for the accident, good communication, explicit protocols and clear chains of command with the rest of their teams.

Homeland Security has a very long way to go to carry out its mission. It not only needs to train and equip as quickly as possible, it has to provide for ongoing research and development, replacements, and maintaining proficiency and accountability. I don't see it happening. Add to that the element of complacency; i.e. the longer we go without another 9/11, the less we focus on being prepared.

To lay people and uninformed professionals, radiation scares the crap out of them. It can't be detected by any of the senses: you don't smell, taste, see, hear or feel it. Fact is, the trained person DOES know how to detect and handle radioactive materials. They give it the utmost respect and get on with the job at hand.

Here are some take home messages (not in priority order) regarding nuclear preparedness:

1. Let's focus on getting first responders fully equipped and trained. Demand more professional involvement and demonstrated readiness.
2. Educate the public with facts. Discourage, even censor, misinformation and strategic omissions. To do otherwise is like deliberately and falsely yelling fire in a theater.
3. Make "energy" part of every school curriculum. Start early.
4. Make it an international felony to violate the collective rules for use of nuclear materials. We need severe, enforceable penalties. The IAEA (International Atomic Energy Agency) is in place but doesn't have requisite power to effectively do its job. Dr. Mohamed El Baradei, the UN nuclear chief for the IAEA, has pointed out the Nuclear Nonproliferation Treaty of the 1960's is in need of revisions to meet modern day challenges. It would require all

countries to give up a degree of autonomy. One of our founding fathers aptly stated, "If we don't hang together, we'll surely hang separately." We simply cannot allow any nation to refuse appropriate inspection by the IAEA.

CHEMICAL

The current mayor of Las Vegas loves to sound off. He and Donald Trump were in the same room for a Las Vegas event. The mayor's wife volunteered:

"Those two men were probably the biggest egos ever, in one room at any time." The Donald is never at a loss for squirrelly ideas, and the mayor apparently feels compelled to compete. Here are three examples:
1. Convert an old downtown federal landmark (a U.S. Post Office) to a mob museum. I'm sure the mayor's photo and exploits will occupy prominent areas (estimated 40 million dollar project).
2. Open a nightspot on Freemont Street with Joe Pesci (the actor) as one of his partners. His former star clients, the Spilotro brothers, wouldn't be available to sweeten the deal. They were beaten to death in an Illinois cornfield…..by prior partners.

3. **Legalize prostitution in Clark County.** Yeah, that would project the right image. Might as well throw in other goodies of an Amsterdam-like city: legalized drugs and euthanasia (not mentioned by the mayor).

The reason I pick on the mayor is because of his cavalier, 'shoot from the hip' statements about other, very serious, topics. He's really not mob-mean(I don't believe he would personally put my head in a vice), but he does like playing to a crowd. For example, he said he would arrest any driver transporting nuclear waste through *HIS city*, and he'd lie down in front of any truck or train carrying such materials. With all due respect, Mr. Mayor, have you looked at the array of chemicals and petroleum products going through *OUR city*? What are you doing to improve the public's safety in that area.

It's not only a Las Vegas problem; it happens all over the United States. We've had chlorine, ammonia, petroleum products and other spills across the country. We've had explosions, fires and loss of life. We had a huge explosion in southern Nevada at a plant manufacturing a component of rocket fuel (perchlorate).

Homeland Security is more focused on terrorist threats using sophisticated materials.

Doesn't it make sense to tighten security for the manufacture and transport of agents we use in everyday commerce? I think it's still relatively easy to get fertilizer and oil to make and transport a bomb similar to the one used by Timothy McVey in Oklahoma.

Let me give you an idea of what healthcare providers should be trained to recognize and treat.

<u>LUNG AGENTS</u>

Chlorine, phosgene, mustard and components of combustion: zinc oxides and oxides of nitrogen, smoke from burning fossil fuels and isocyanates/polyurethane foams…and myriad combinations. These agents may act in various ways. They can cause direct irritation and/or damage to lung tissue. They can act on mechanisms that control or affect the ability of the lungs to expand and contract. They may cause a combination of these effects.

In some instances we have no specific treatments or antidotes. All we can do is support the patient with oxygen, fluids, antibiotics, pain management and tide them over, with the hope of allowing the body to heal itself; partially or completely.

VESICANTS

Also referred to as blister agents; agents that irritate the skin and body orifices. Phosgene, mustard and Lewisite are examples. Treatment is primarily supportive and symptoms depend on the severity and length of exposure. Secondary infections may occur, and pre-existing medical conditions may worsen.

BLOOD AGENTS (CYANOGENS)

Hydrogen Cyanide affects the ability of cells to use oxygen, while Cyanogen Chloride affects the central nervous system, heart muscle and certain chemical receptor sites in the body. Depending on the concentration and speed of inhalation, it can cause difficulty in breathing, convulsions (seizures) or irregular rhythms…resulting in death. These agents can be treated with specific antidotes such as Amyl Nitrite, Sodium Nitrite, and Sodium Thiosulfate—as well as supportive therapy like oxygen, fluids, attention to airway, circulation, breathing, removal from toxic environment and decontamination.

Aside from having enough trained people, do we have the equipment, medicines, designated staging areas and clear protocols for communication? I say, definitely not!

NERVE AGENTS

These chemicals interfere with nerve impulse transmission. Two general groups are the Carbamates and Organophosphates... commonly used as household and commercial insecticides. In general, they cause over-stimulation of organ systems, or block signals to body organs. We do have specific antidotes for these agents.

Sarin, released in the subway system in Japan, demonstrated how easy it is to frighten and injure. Tabun and Soman are nerve agents that could be used in a similar fashion.

The important message relative to chemical, biologic and nuclear agents is that we do understand what these agents can do, and we know our capabilities for protection, isolation, decontamination and treatment. However, no matter how well we prepare with training and physical resources, it's obvious a determined terrorist effort could overwhelm what we've allegedly put in place for protection and treatment. We must continually do research and development, training and equipping response teams, educate and enlist the public's *eyes and ears*.

We must move to eliminate internal and global turf battles. We either unite now, or pay a horrible price later. It means universal inventories and tracking systems for all materials capable of causing harm. I'm not very optimistic about the world being ready to set aside special interests for the common good, but I'll support any and all efforts in those directions.

BACTERIOLOGIC

Infectious agents, like chemical and nuclear, are fairly well understood by the scientific community. For those in the trenches doing daily surveillance and treatments, it means having a high index of suspicion for anything resembling departure from the expected or the routine. The first responders don't have to have all the details for any specific agent, but they have to be very familiar with general policies and procedures. They have to have quick access to diagnostic laboratory facilities, a reasonable supply of appropriate equipment, related materials and therapeutic agents. The chains of command have to be clearly delineated. We can never become complacent. Practice drills need to be practiced often enough to ensure all personnel are ready if called to action. With this in mind, let's look at historical facts and scenarios.

Dr. Dennis G. Maki, M.D., Head, Section of Infectious Diseases, University of Wisconsin

Medical School, made a wonderful presentation at a medical meeting in Las Vegas, November 3, 2001. I present portions of his handout (my comments in parenthesis).

"The world is confronted in the early 21st Century by the specter of biologic warfare, or more likely, bioterrorism. The use of infectious agents as weapons by governments or terrorist groups is not a new concept. During World War II, the Japanese government weaponized anthrax, plague and cholera organisms, which they dropped on Chinese cities. (None of those responsible faced trial for war crimes...why?)

The potential for large-scale bioterrorism in our lifetime has been brought to fruition by the knowledge that during the past 50 years the Soviet Union has maintained a huge and sophisticated biologic warfare research program, hidden in every ministry of its government. At its height during the 1980's, it encompassed 65,000 scientists and support personnel, and weaponized many tons of anthrax spores, small pox virus, and a variety of other pathogens. With the dissolution of the Soviet economy, numerous scientists and support personnel in their program were recruited by countries that support international terrorism, such as Iraq and Libya, among the worldwide dozen or so known to have bioweapon capacity.

It is most likely that, if bioweapons are used, whether against military personnel or civilians, it will be by individual terrorist groups rather than by governments that could be implicated and suffer devastating retaliation. There are good reasons to fear the al Qaeda group may have access to biologic weapons they are planning to use. The most likely agents to be used are anthrax and smallpox, both of which have probably been available on the world black market in weaponized forms.

The best overall protection against bioterrorism will be an unrelenting effort on the part of all governments of the world to root out and totally eliminate terrorism in every form."

Dr. Maki then went on to give a long and shameful history of bioterrorism:

- 1346: Tartars catapult plaque-infected corpses into besieged city of Kaffa….? source of Europe's Black Death.
- 1710: Russians did same against Sweden.
- 1500's: Conquistadors gave Incas smallpox-laden clothes.
- 1760's: British gave American Indians smallpox-laden blankets.

WW II: Japanese dropped anthrax, plague and cholera organisms on Chinese cities. 10,000 prisoners died in biologic experiments (Americans among them).

1943-72: U.S. B.W. research at Ft. Detrick, Maryland. Anthrax, Plague, Botulism, Tularemia, Q Fever, Brucella and others. Our programs were aimed at defensive solutions.

1958-present: Soviet Union's huge BW program. Anthrax, Smallpox, Plague, Tularemia, Ebola Virus and others.

1979: Sverdlosk; BW facility in USSR produced tons of Anthrax spores each year in a fine dust form for weaponization (over 30 tons in continuous storage), genetically engineered to be resistant to penicillin and tetracycline antibiotics. There was an accidental release due to a faulty filter. Less than 100 grams of spores was estimated in the release. It caused cattle to die beyond 30 miles downwind. 96 human cases with 76 deaths over 44 days, despite the recognition of the outbreak within 1 week. The government attempted to cover it up by saying it resulted from contaminated meat. Of note, BORIS YELTSIN was governor of Sverdlosk at the time.

1970's: Laos "yellow rain". Not sure of the agent. Maybe mycotoxin?

1972: Biologic and Toxin Weapons Convention (BWC); 140 countries signatories, including USSR and Iraq.

1984: Rajneeshees cult spread S. typhimurium organism onto salad bars in Dallas and Oregon. 751 cases of enteritis.

1995: Japanese Aum Shinriko cult release Sarin gas into Tokyo subway. 5000 exposed; 12 deaths.

2000: Countries considered to have active BW programs: Russia, Iraq, Iran, Lybia, N. Korea, Syria, China. Could be many times this number.

BIOTERRORISM – NOT IF, BUT WHEN?

Dr. Maki continued with common fallacies about Biologic Warfare/
Biologic Terrorism:
- It won't happen.
- Feds in suits will arrive to save the day.
- Our superior public health system and medical care will prove effective.

THE REALITY IS:

- **U.S. has many enemies, including rogue states and terrorist groups unaffiliated with any single country. Many terrorists willing to die to inflict great damage.**
- **Technology for BW/BT is readily available, as well as huge quantities of weaponized BW agents. We cannot account for USSR stockpiles, nor Iraq, or other countries programs.**
- **No warning likely.**
- **Cases unlikely to be diagnosed promptly.**
- **Most cities and hospitals not prepared.**
- **Cases will overwhelm healthcare system and Public Health/Federal resources.**
- **Massive panic highly likely.**
- **Many people will die.**

By looking at the reality bullets, we can determine what has to be done in order to deter and prepare for the worst. It has become a fact of life, and most agree, it will take a full commitment for as long as it takes—which probably means forever.

Las Vegas, like other tourist and business destinations, will require more resources and training as compared to smaller, rural areas. We have approximately 40 million visitors a year. Just one nut and a threat of blowing himself/

herself up in the lobby of a major hotel, could seriously impact the number one industry of the state. Or, as Tom Clancy portrayed in one of his books, a terrorist could attend one of our major conventions and distribute several aerosol cans around the meeting areas. Timing devices on the cans could be set to release invisible amounts of Plague or Anthrax. The exposed people become carriers as well as targets. They carry it back to their communities.

Pneumonic forms of Plague can spread from person to person, whereas Anthrax will not. The public panic and social disruption is about as difficult to comprehend as our gross national deficit. We, like the rest of the country and world, have to make lifelong commitments for the following, as expressed by Dr. Maki.

- Vigorous international condemnation/isolation of countries with <u>Offensive</u> BW programs.
- Consistent and more effective international inspections.
- Highly sensitive "biodetectors."
- Ample stockpile of critical vaccines and anti-infectives.
- Research to develop better vaccines and therapeutics.

- **More rapid and reliable diagnostic techniques.**
- **Greatly strengthened national, state and local programs to deal with possible BT/BW.**
- **Better prepared physicians, other healthcare workers and hospitals.**
- **Better networks for communication and reporting.**
- **A strong national resolve and defense.**

I would add that we have to educate our children from early on, and our adults as soon as possible. They are the frontline eyes and ears. Just as we educate to be wary of strangers and aware of one's surroundings, we must educate for the climate of terrorism.

I would caution against getting hung up with semantics and emotionalism. For example, using the word profiling drives many people into knee-jerk hysterics, pontificating about infringement of constitutional rights or embarking on vigilantism.

Think for a moment, how do I, as a physician, go about making a diagnosis? I take a history, do a physical exam, add some lab data and evaluate the sum of it all against "profiles" of most likely causes for the presenting signs and symptoms. Is this very different from the process of screening for people intent on doing harm?

If we selected someone for closer scrutiny <u>solely</u> on the basis of their looking like a member of an ethnic group, I agree it would be pushing the bounds of constitutional privacy. However, I see no problem with using ethnicity as one factor for the process of solving a puzzle. It is similar to my taking a person for further study because they present with a fever, rash and swollen glands. Whether we like it or not, a profile of factors can legitimately raise the index of suspicion…..for medical solutions, or to root out persons intent on doing us harm.

We should be ready and willing to provide justification for our actions. For example, I should be able to unequivocally justify ordering imaging or lab tests, for the purpose of pursuing a diagnosis.

The stakes are too high to err on the side of being timid. I'll be happy to apologize if it turned out I was overzealous or misled. We must discuss our ethical options and pressing needs, and arrive at workable solutions.

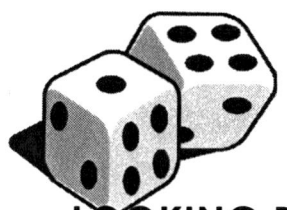 # CHAPTER IX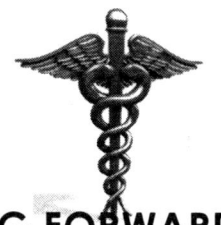

LOOKING BACK AND WONDERING FORWARD

Blessed with good health and a long, varied, productive career, I enjoy reminiscing about cases and scenarios. I also stroke my chin and wonder about tomorrow's conundrums.

One of the saddest trends in medicine has been the disappearance of old fashioned, Marcus Welby-type family physicians. They're now called primary care physicians, and patients are frequently referred to as clients or units. Since 1997, there has been a 50 percent drop in medical graduates choosing to go into family practice specialty training. The big money and attraction appears to be in medical management and selected specialties. The relatively new afternoon TV show, THE DOCTORS, has a plastic surgeon, a pediatrician, an ob-gyn and an emergency room physician as panelists....no family physician; why?

The University of Nevada School of Medicine (UNSOM) has done a good job in getting more physicians into rural communities but a great need still exists. A young physician may be willing to take on the challenges of 24/7 coverage for a small community, but what about the needs of his family? Can the community provide opportunities if the spouse has a career of his/her own? Are there people in the community who can provide stimulating social interaction? This is not an elitist question. It's a fact of life.

People who have been fortunate enough to experience higher education, and all that goes with it, tend to look for groups of like-minded people. Will the physician in a small community get enough free time to enjoy his/her family, and recharge the batteries?

In addition to lifestyles, there are questions of money and respect. Small communities usually hold their "Doc" in high regard…unless he/she is a complete jerk. Big city colleague-specialists, and patients, are prone to treat the family physician as a lesser professional. The status question is compounded by lower reimbursements schedules.

There was a temporary increase in the primary care workforce in the 1990's. This was in response to federal incentive policies and funding efforts. However, specialization has once again dominated postgraduate choices among M.D. medical school graduates. It may be time to reorient our system to primary care… as expressed in an editorial in American Family Physician, October 15, 2003 (page 1494). My comments are added in parentheses.

"The policy options for reorienting our health care system to primary care have been on the table for more than a decade and include the following:

- Reimbursement that facilitates and rewards continuous, patient-centered, comprehensive, compassionate and coordinated care. Reimbursement that reflects the special challenge of primary care, fostering patient-focused continuity and maximizing quality and safety. Reimbursement that promotes team practice and offers patients the expertise and training of each member rather than having them compete to fill the same rolls.
- Developing and supporting information systems and decision-support tools that help primary care physicians improve the quality of primary health care, and to know when it is time to involve subspecialists.
- Using state licensing laws, population health needs assessments, and funding to shape an appropriate workforce.

- **Explicit subsidies for training programs that produce primary care physicians.**
- **Expansion of loan forgiveness for primary care physicians.**
- **Adequate support for practice-based research and primary care health services research.**
- **Measuring and rewarding effective care, especially preventive care services.**
- **Supporting better connections between primary health care, public health, mental health and subspecialty services.**

Failure to find the will to change is a path to increasingly poor outcomes, escalating costs, and the dismantling of primary care infrastructures that will take decades to rebuild. There appears to be some resurgence of optimism, or at least urgency, for offering health care coverage for everyone in the United States (It was a hot-button issue in the 2008 national election). If this latest effort develops momentum among the public and policy makers, it may offer an opportunity to develop a health care system that is more appropriately oriented to primary care, and that supports the needed workforce to deliver its promise.

Current trends have been to use physician extenders such as physician assistants and nurse practitioners. The main argument given is that they provide easier and cheaper accessibility; healthcare extenders work cheaper and train quicker...but there may be quality drawbacks.

Pharmacy chains in Nevada have set up walk-in clinics staffed by physician extenders. A licensed physician in Nevada is legally permitted to hire 3 extenders. With the current entrepreneurial emphasis on easy access and big volumes, I foresee problems with quality oversight. Everyone is happy until preventable errors start popping up....and they will, in my opinion.

Family physicians must become engaged in working through their own organizations, and working with consumer groups to educate the public and policy makers about the need for immediate action. Most family physicians I know say they're too burdened making ends meet to get involved. They claim mounting paperwork, regulations and government intrusions shrink their ability to do anything other than looking after patients, and family. If they don't get involved, others will make the decisions for them.

The United States leads the world in many ways: militarily, economically (debatable) and in health care spending. Health care spending of $1.7 trillion per year should be sufficient to place the United States in the lead in health and health care outcomes. However, we find ourselves behind nearly all of our nation's industrialized peers with regard to health outcomes. We currently face another primary care workforce crisis that is compounded by increased diversion of medical school graduates into subspecialties. We appear to lack the political will to reorient our system to primary care and to provide coverage and access to health care for all Americans."

On a personal note: after 13 years of old-fashioned, home/office, family practice (1960–1973), I decided on a career change, primarily because I could not find anyone to help with my 18-20 hour days. I moved to Nevada and added another specialty to my certification as a family physician; The American Board of Occupational and Environmental Medicine (ABOEM). I continued to be a member of the Nevada Academy of Family Physicians (NAFP). I attended more NAFP meetings than most family physicians in southern Nevada, including the annual ski meetings at Tahoe; a wonderful session for education, recreation and networking. I can attest to the fact that few family practitioners in southern Nevada, percentage-wise, belong to the NAFP, and even less regularly attend their meetings or get involved in the policy forming or political process. When Nevada physicians mobilized to initiate medical malpractice reform in 2004, family practitioners, pediatricians, dermatologists and psychiatrists were notably absent in vocal participation and monetary support. The high-priced specialties, with the high malpractice premiums, like obstetrics/gynecology, neurosurgery, anesthesia, orthopedics and general surgery gave the most money and time.

Newcomers to southern Nevada frequently ask me whom they can go to for medical care. I have increasing difficulty in processing their requests….for several reasons:

1. Unrealistic patient expectations lead to embarrassments…or worse.
2. Difficult to find family physicians who still practice the 4-A's: Affordable, Affable, Available and Accessible.
3. Medical-legal ramifications. I could become a defendant by making a recommendation.

My getting elected Chief of Staff for University Medical Center in 1982 (the only not-for-profit teaching hospital in southern Nevada) was helped by mobilizing members of the Family Practice Department. That Department had never had a true representative for family practitioners, and when I finished my two-year term, they have never again gotten adequate representation.

The teaching hospital continually complains about competing for paying patients. It's not rocket science…go out of your way to attract the "gatekeepers", i.e. family practitioners and internists. Make sure the hospital is doctor friendly and patient friendly by paying attention to parking, record keeping, bed availability, continuous dialogue, respect, inclusion, and a full spectrum of support services. The hospital stewards have to be committed to minimizing politics, turf battles and special interests.

There are signs of optimism for those of us interacting with tomorrow's physicians. The newer graduates are dedicated, well trained, enthusiastic and generally ready for the complex challenges that await them. For sure, a miniscule number can be recognized for being committed to money more than principles. Thankfully, in my experience, these are the exceptions. (I am talking primarily about M.D. physicians, since I do not have significant interaction with DO's).

Just compare the overall public's perception of M.D. healthcare providers to those of politicians, lawyers, corporate directors, media spinners, auditors…and even the clergy. The medical profession is not perfect, but they stand very high by comparison to other vocations, using any number of yardsticks.

For newer medical colleagues, and lay people reading this book, I'd like to outline the post World War II route to medical practice, and point out changes that have occurred along the way.

My generation, graduating college in the 50's, took a 4-year pre-medical program and applied to a 4-year medical college. After 8 years, the medical graduate would have a choice of doing a 1-year rotating internship, applying for a medical license and starting practice, or they could choose specialty training. The year's internship consisted of 3-month rotations in surgery, internal medicine, obstetrics/gynecology and pediatrics. Somewhere in those rotations one might get brief exposures to ophthalmology, dermatology, psychiatry.

Some decided to go into specialty training programs called residencies, which lasted from 2 to 4 years. Completion of a residency, and the specialty exam, qualified that person as a *board certified specialist* in their chosen field. A specialist was usually in their early 30's by the time they started a licensed medical practice. The MD's have largely bypassed the intern option and now go directly into specialty (residency) programs upon graduation from medical school. Family Practice is now a 3-year, board certified specialty. Neurosurgery takes 7 years of training after medical school. A resident usually starts around $30,000 per year. The instructors for resident clinical training are either full time teaching physicians, or practicing physicians with part-time teaching appointments.

The "making of a doctor" is a long, demanding and expensive process. In this day and age, many medical school graduates get their diplomas with $50,000 to $150,000 of debt. Most current medical school classes are 50 percent, or more, female. I had 3 women in a class of 52, back in the 1950's. I have also noted a marked increase in foreign-born (first generation Americans) coming into the medical workforce. Ethnic and gender changes have grown out of social upheavals, world and local political conditions, economic factors and media "stimuli". The changes have brought pluses and minuses. Wars have created new techniques and procedures, but have also stressed and adversely influenced our healthcare system. I believe the general public and politicians have no appreciation of the needs and magnitude for follow-up care of the casualties of the second Gulf war.

Graduates of foreign medical schools have their own hurdles. I would have to follow similar paths if I went to practice in their country. They have to take English language and medical proficiency exams, enter U. S. training programs (usually 3-year minimum) and pass licensing examinations to practice in the United States. The forces of supply and demand bring about periodic changes in training and licensing requirements; i.e. requirements loosen up when we need more bodies, and tighten up with the reverse.

Gaming of licensing rules applies to allied health professionals: LPN's (lesser-trained, licensed practical nurses) or nurse assistants replacing RN's (registered nurses who've completed 4-year college programs). Nurse anesthetists replacing M.D. anesthesiologists. States claiming shortages of anesthesia personnel have dropped the discretionary federal requirement for physician supervision of nurse anesthetists (approximately 15 states to date). The U.S. continually moves toward cheaper and quicker ways to fill the healthcare body shortage. You need to judge the end product. Are you satisfied with the results? If not, are you willing to pay more and demand more?

One case doesn't prove a hell of a lot, but it does stick in my memory because of the players. Do you remember President Bill Clinton's mother? She was a nurse anesthetist in Arkansas. She was allegedly responsible for at least two deaths (one was allegedly due to incorrectly placing an endotracheal tube). The allegations were never denied and the case did not come to a trial. The Arkansas official charged with deciding if it should proceed to trial, had been appointed to his job by Governor Bill Clinton; at the very least, a perceived conflict of interest. You can't have "foxes in the henhouse watching out for the chickens".

What are some of the things we need if we're seriously looking to expand affordable, accessible healthcare?

<u>HEALTH CARE PROVIDERS AND LEGISLATORS</u>

1. We need uniform federal standards.
2. Clarify rules and regulations to eliminate escape routes for transgressors.
3. Impose mandatory penalties that truly discourage wrongdoing.
4. Malpractice reform along the provisions of California's MICRA.
5. A single board in every state to license physicians (and allied health professionals).

6. A collective will that puts special interests secondary to the greater good. The 'players' need to move up to the plate.

THE CONSUMER-PATIENT

If you didn't get a good set of genes from your parents, you may have to work harder to minimize your health risks. Don't smoke, drink in moderation, keep your body mass within reasonable levels, exercise, be positive and productive with activities of daily living. Become educated to realistic, proven, medical facts and look for a good healthcare provider.

You should now understand what those initials after a doctor's name stand for. Check for references from the County and State medical societies, health groups and residents within the community. If your providers can't communicate effectively and/or are not available (personally or with adequate backup coverage), keep looking. Consider second opinions, especially with non-urgent problems.

Have annual checkups and learn to recognize signs and symptoms requiring further investigation. Know what is reasonable and indicated for your age, sex and special needs. Don't look the other way just because someone else is paying for it.

If your provider is willing to do creative billing or alter insurance papers, then how trustworthy are they in providing recommendations or direct care?

Health food claims and food supplements are essentially unregulated by the Food and Drug Administration (FDA). Consider their claims suspect until proven otherwise by reputable scientific studies. It's tragic when such claims raise false hopes and squander precious resources. It becomes even more tragic when such activities interfere with, or detract from, legitimate medical help.

When you get a bill from a hospital, or provider, don't plunk down the co-pay unless you're totally satisfied with the statements. Wait until the insurance carriers deliver what they owe, and critically review all statements. If there are questions or discrepancies not adequately addressed by the providers, seek out state or local Ombudspersons to investigate and mediate.

As with any other game, if you don't learn and apply the rules, your chances of winning will be small indeed. Try and tilt the odds in your favor, whenever 'you roll the dice'.

REFLECTIONS OF A TIMELESS JOURNEY

(From a St. Rose Hospital publication, Las Vegas, Nevada)
The adventure of life is to learn.
The purpose of life is to grow.
The nature of life is to change.
The challenge of life is to overcome.
The essence of life is to care.
The opportunity of life is to serve.
The secret of life is to dare.
The spice of life is to befriend.
The beauty of life is to give.
Author – Unknown

THE END

Made in the USA